things you, can't ask yer mom

things you, can't ask yer mom

**LIZZY HADFIELD &
LINDSEY HOLLAND**

K

An Hachette UK Company
www.hachette.co.uk

First published in Great Britain in 2021
by Kyle Books,
an imprint of Octopus Publishing Group
Limited
Carmelite House
50 Victoria Embankment
London EC4Y 0DZ
www.octopusbooks.com

This edition published in 2021.

ISBN: 978 0 85783 964 0

Distributed in the US by Hachette Book
Group, 1290 Avenue of the Americas,
4th and 5th Floors, New York, NY 10104

Distributed in Canada by Canadian
Manda Group, 664 Annette St., Toronto,
Ontario, Canada M6S 2C8

Publisher: Joanna Copestick
Editorial Director: Judith Hannam
Senior Commissioning Editor:
Louise McKeever
Design: Rosamund Saunders
Copy-editor: Liz Marvin
Production: Caroline Alberti

A Cataloguing in Publication record
for this title is available from the
British Library

Printed and bound in Great Britain

10 9 8 7 6 5 4 3 2 1

The FSC® label means that materials
used for the product have been
responsibly sourced.

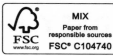

MIX
Paper from
responsible sources
FSC
www.fsc.org
FSC® C104740

*This is more of an apology
than a dedication, to both of
our incredible moms. We're
sorry you're going to have
to read about our sex lives.
We love you very much.*

Contents

Introduction

Writing a book was not something either of us imagined
we would ever do. But then again, neither was starting
a podcast, getting to travel the globe as best friends, or
sharing our dreadful one-night stand stories with the world.
But if this has taught us anything, it's that life is unexpected
and you just have to roll with it all anyway.

Our friendship has always been about sharing our highs and
lows, and supporting one another no matter what—finding
the balance between tough love when it's needed, never
meeting the other with judgment, and always being there to
pick up the pieces without an "I told you so" in sight.

Our podcast even came about from one of those moments
in life when you suddenly find yourself truly on your knees.

One evening in May 2019, while deeply enthralled in an episode of *Ozark*, Lindsey's phone lit up. Though Lindsey wouldn't interrupt her evenings to look at her phone for many people, Lizzy is, of course, one of the exceptions. The text read: "I have a question, and you are 100 percent the best person to ask for this. Have you ever given someone a blow job when you have tonsillitis? If anyone in the world has, it'll be you."

Firstly, charming! Secondly, yes, she had come to the right person. The answer was yes, Lindsey had indeed, and a) it causes pain and b) we assume a mix of bacteria that would rival any antibiotic. Lindsey replied and said #thingsyoucantaskyermom.

So this is how tonsillitis and blow jobs led us to create our podcast *Things You Can't Ask Yer Mum*, which we have built into a safe space where we talk through our own experiences of love, grief, self-doubt, and everything in between, in the hope that listeners will feel connected to themselves and to us. We wanted to show that you are absolutely not alone in your feelings, thoughts, or medical scenarios (just wait until you hear about the time Lindsey's sexual antics resulted in her hands swelling up to three times their usual size).

And so the hashtag that launched a thousand podcast episodes (not quite, but you get the gist) has transformed again—into our first book. A place for us to write down those pearls of wisdom for all of you, so many of which have been inspired by our audience and the questions we have been asked over the years. It's made us realize how similar everyone's thoughts and feelings can be, despite the specific differences in everyone's circumstances. Which certainly helped us to feel less alone too! Our experiences are recorded from two different perspectives, through tears, beers, and laughing until no noise would leave our bodies. Next, we wanted to extend our beloved *Things You Can't Ask Yer Mum* community to the page, so we could give you something physical to provide comfort, laughs, and the advice and learnings we all seek at one stage in our life or another.

> "We built our podcast and this book off the back of true love, the kind of true love you can't find in a romantic partner, only in a true friend."

We are different in how we deal with things, which is what makes this book the equivalent of the varied advice you look for when you decide which message group is the place to share your woes instead of seeking just one person's take on a situation. Lizzy likes to write everything down, explore every possibility and angle, and discuss the same topic over and over until we can speak of it no more. Lindsey, on the other hand, likes to burn sage on a full moon and make decisions on impulse (if the moon allows, of course). The differences between us are what have made our friendship so balanced; it's how we complement one another and learn from each other, and this is what we want to impart to you. The chance to see it all in black and white, to return to this book over and over again when you need it (as per Lizzy's coping mechanisms) and also to understand that life is taking you on the path that is meant for you, no matter how scary it feels at times (as per Lindsey's impulses, which have always landed her on her feet, and sometimes even when it wasn't a full moon!).

After all, opposites attract, as they say. We built our podcast and this book off the back of true love, the kind of true love you can't find in a romantic partner, only in a true friend. We've weathered some huge storms together and we'd like to think that this book will reassure you in times of self-doubt, give you hope when you're gripped by heartbreak, and be a best buddy to lean on when everything starts to go wrong. And most importantly, we know you're likely to follow your heart with all of your decisions, so if we're the friend you text saying, "Thank you for your advice, I went and did the total opposite," we will still be here without a shred of judgment (maybe an eye roll, at most).

'To provide comfort, laughs and the advice and learnings we all seek.'

Each chapter of this book offers two sides to the story. A section written by Lindsey and one by Lizzy. We will discuss certain topics together at certain points, or offer you some practical advice. But the main thing we want you to be able to take away is two different experiences of each part of life.

An important note to end on: HOW you read this book will be the deciding factor in if you are more Camp Lizzy or Camp Lindsey. A book read by Lindsey looks like it has been through the washing machine, pages turned down, dog-eared and spine broken. A book read by Lizzy looks exactly the same as it did when the first page was read—completely pristine. So either make a mental note of the pages you want to return to without defacing them or write every thought and feeling you have in every bit of white space and fold down every page. The point is that this book is for YOU, whoever you are, whatever you identify with, and whatever point you're at in life. Enjoy it, savor it, return to it, and maybe don't lend it to your mom ...

CHAPTER 1

Friendship

We have to start the book here, with friendship, as so many great things would never have happened if we hadn't met and become friends. We have been friends for eight years now, after meeting through work during London Fashion Week (we were actually sat in a bar, so it wasn't quite as glamorous as that might sound!). Both hailing from the north of England, we instantly got on.

Lizzy was in Manchester then and Lindsey moved to London from Preston after a big breakup (which we will of course be discussing later in this book) so, over the next four years, our friendship grew slowly, though it became stronger in the six months before Lizzy's own breakup. Firstly it withstood a trip to Copenhagen in January, where Lindsey complained about the cold *endlessly,* only to then instantly complain she was too hot as soon as she was back inside. That first trip we ever did together was filled with laughter and a new appreciation for Miss Holland's diva alter ego that specifically comes out on planes, at extreme temperatures, or when she has to carry a heavy bag.

Later that same year we went to Berlin, where Lizzy first opened up to Lindsey about her own relationship doubts. This was the beginning of the end of her first long-term love. It was the first time Lizzy had ever spoken openly to someone about it; she'd been trying to tell herself that everything was fine. She began by saying, "And I know it's totally normal to feel this way ..." only to see Lindsey's face tell her everything she needed to know. In the most balanced and gentle way, that slowly lets someone stare reality in the face, Lindsey kindly put it into words: it wasn't normal; the feelings likely wouldn't go away and there was more waiting for Lizzy out there. It was the beginning of a whole new connection between us, where we knew we would always be met with honesty and love, no matter what the issue was.

Lizzy's relationship finally ended about six months later, after which she moved to London and our friendship flourished even more. In the years since then, there have been countless trips filled with amazing memories— booking flights to the wrong airport in the Caribbean, Lizzy crying all night on a drunken New York night out and ruining Lindsey's silk blouse with her tears, and some excellent wing-woman moments from Lindsey. Plus plenty of amazing moments closer to home, too. We have held each other through relationship problems, breakups, grief, and the career highs and lows that seem relentless at times. We have learned so much from one another and very regularly say to each other, "GOOD HEAVENS! Imagine the state I would be in if I didn't have you." We know how lucky we are to have a friendship like this, so in this chapter we will share with you how we built it and nurtured it, as well as, by way of contrast, the not-so-successful experiences we have had in other friendships over the years.

"Friendships can be hard work; they can be testing, and the good ones are often hard to find."

Letters between best friends

Dear Lindsey,

To say that I would be lost without you would be an understatement. I have lost count of how many times I have messaged you asking for advice about one thing or another. We haven't gone a day without speaking in years now and I really hope we don't any time soon (please don't block me no matter how many times I ask you the same questions!).

You have taught me so, so much. The power of unwavering loyalty and the respect that deserves. The importance of going the extra mile for people without expecting anything in return. The different ways you can always offer an ear to someone—a shoulder to cry on, a phone number to leave a very long voicemail to. You are always there for people in a way I admire so much and anyone who knows you personally will nod along as they read this because at some point they too will have been on the receiving end of your selflessness.

However, you have a very large ego as it is so now I must take you down a peg or two! You are truly a nightmare to travel with at times. How many times have I given up the window seat on the plane? Listened to you complain about being even one degree above or below your desired temperature? Carried the heavier bag because I could sense a hissy fit coming on at a time it would be best to keep it together? And yet I can safely say, I wouldn't change any of it and there is no one else I would rather travel the world with. (But I would like the window seat just ONCE!)

We have built a friendship on so much mutual respect and effort. It's been made easier by the fact we are both very, very funny and give one another the appreciation our jokes deserve. But I will always be grateful for the number of times you have been at the end of the phone for me. Have hugged me on the couch as I sobbed over a broken heart. Have offered the same advice over and over again when I need to talk through the same problem one more time. How many times you have helped my six-pack along by making me laugh so much. Have come and just sat in my house to keep me company on the days I needed it. And have planned trips and getaways when you could sense how much I was struggling with something.

We both know exactly what to say to each other and when. How to comfort one another when the response "Yeah, I'm OK" really means we are NOT OK and are in fact sat at home feeling like our life is crashing down around us. Sometimes I will be on the brink of some sort of breakdown and my phone will light up with a "Lizzy-loo, how are you doing?" It's like we are in sync.

Thank you for everything; I think you're most likely my soul mate and I am just sorry I don't fancy you.

Lizzy xx

Dear Lizzy,

There is nobody quite like you, Lizzy—a woman still in her twenties with the wisdom of someone who has lived a lifetime. You show it in your ability to be pragmatic at times when I'm at my most impulsive. And it comes out in your softness and equally the hard edge that surrounds you when you need to protect yourself and those around you—i.e., me. I have never met someone so unassuming in their intelligence, kindness, or beauty.

I have loved traveling the world with you. (Though thanks for throwing me and my high-maintenance ways under the bus, buddy.) You have taught me how to slow down, how to take things more softly, and even how to accept myself and those around me, no matter what the issue. And regardless of the Leo inside me wanting to tear things down.

You can't cook. But you're getting better. You've not managed to poison me yet but you have made me eat dinner from the floor after you cooked it then threw it all over the kitchen by accident. I have a video of this which shall continue to be shared as a biannual reminder.

Our friendship is my favorite thing. We never pass judgment on one another but give each other our honest opinions, good or hard, filled with love and support.

Countless times we have sobbed on each other's shoulders over one heartbreak or another and I wouldn't want a soggy collar or mascara-stained silk shirt from anybody else.
You calm down my fire and I'm pissed because it's making me a better person (I already thought I was quite good).

Love,

Linds xx

Lizzy on **Friendships**

I truly believe that friendships are the foundation of so much happiness in life and should therefore be given as much priority as a romantic relationship. When I look around at my friends, I realize that they have facilitated more personal growth and understanding than any man I have had in my life and have always done so with the utmost patience and understanding. The way women understand other women is something I will always be in awe of.

But, that being said, friendships can be hard work; they can be testing, and the good ones are often hard to find. As you get older and have a stronger sense of yourself, it can be harder to find yourself among like-minded people. Especially when we feel that everyone has their friendship groups sorted already. What makes those bonds so strong can also make them seen intimidating and impenetrable if you're stood on the outside.

We learn this feeling as early as elementary school, when we become aware of cliques, the concept of popularity, and how important it is to feel like you have your own group around you to provide that vital sense of acceptance and belonging. I will never forget the first day of junior high when I struck my initial bond with my friend Katie, who is still one of my closest friends. We were both hovering on the outskirts of the friendship between the two "popular girls," neither of us being fully accepted into the already very tight-knit pairing. One day on the locker corridor, we found ourselves in fits of laughter together over something and from that moment a friendship was made. It was so exhilarating. I was more excited to go to school after that and to make plans (via our moms, who in turn have remained very good friends) for the weekends. It was literally life-changing as it was the start of a friendship that has been in my life from that day on. The intimidating and self-conscious feeling of being on the outside of the initial popular group compared to the warmth and happiness of being on the inside of my own group (albeit just the two of us!) is a distinction I think we all learn early on in life and one that stays with us throughout adulthood.

Lots of good comes from this process. When making the effort to meet new people as an adult, you begin to learn more about what your "type" is in a friendship. We all know the feeling of meeting someone and just thinking, "Thank you, but no." They can be perfectly polite and kind and it really is nothing they have done, they are just not your person. And chances are you won't be theirs either. In my experience, that moment when you first recognize the feeling I've just described marks an empowering shift between wanting to make *any* friendship work—such as in the early high school days when you're all thrown in together—to realizing you get a choice in the matter and can actually bypass the people to whom you don't want to give your time. When you start to find the good ones, if you put the right amount of energy into those friendships and give them time and love to make them grow, you will be onto a winning combination.

Onto the matter of actually meeting these good ones. As an adult, this can feel tricky. Throughout school and university, we are thrown together with groups of new people with whom we have guaranteed common ground—you are often from similar backgrounds, might have grown up in the same place, are studying the same thing—and you don't have to find time for each other because your daily life revolves around shared activities. While you still have those outsider moments, it's easier to find your group because there are a lot of people in the same place to choose from. As you slip into the terrifying realm of adulthood, you see what a privilege that was at about the same time you realize it probably won't happen that way again and now it will take some effort to meet new people. A ball ache, I know.

I think it's a generally accepted idea that when you're single and wanting to date, you're open to new things, saying yes, and you have an invisible green light on that says: "YES, I WOULD LIKE TO MEET YOU" (maybe not in capitals, that would depend on how long it was since you last had sex). I think it can work the same way with friendships too (not the sex part), when you turn on a green light that says: "YES, I WANT TO MEET NEW PEOPLE." Now, I think I may need to go and invent these lights so we can have them in a literal sense, but in the meantime the equivalent is to say yes to as much as possible—and be vulnerable.

As I get older, I see the importance of being vulnerable more and more. Say to someone, "I would love to come out with you and your friends this weekend if it wouldn't be intrusive and you think we might get on. I would love to meet some new people." You have to be prepared to accept their response and trust their judgment on the matter, but with that mindset you only need a small handful of friends as a gateway to more friendships. Equally, make sure you are making the effort to connect people, too. As with lots of things, you get back what you put in—and connecting people you know will get on will make your and their life much easier when it comes to making new friends.

> *"Showing up and truly being yourself can be scary; if you suffer rejection, when you are doing your best, it's the ultimate let down."*

Vulnerability is so important within the friendships you forge, too, just as with any relationship. It can be very scary but for me, being honest and open with my friends has been the stepping-stone to me being a bit better at being vulnerable overall. When you are true to yourself and learn that doing that can make you feel safe and accepted, it creates such a healthy space for open conversations and trust. Though it's also important to remember that not every friendship in your life has to be the same: some involve speaking every day and sharing all aspects of your life, others only really exist once a month over a wine, some even less frequently than that. But no matter what form the friendship takes, the thing is that you do what you can to give the other person what they need in that moment, with the trust that they are going to do the same for you. That's the give and take of being vulnerable with someone and it's joyful when you find yourself with a handful of friendships like that in your life.

That said, showing up and truly being yourself can be scary; if you suffer rejection when you are being authentic and doing your best, it's the ultimate let down. Or at the time it is, anyway—in the long run it will be the best thing that can happen. Because if you have that feeling over and over again in a friendship, you need to be able to recognize it and act, because that is a major sign of a toxic friendship. Though removing yourself from it is often just as painful as extracting yourself from the throes of a toxic romance, with the heartbreak and all. Often it takes a while to see the negative effects that someone you count as a friend is having on you. My experiences with friendships that have turned toxic have always involved a slow burn of self-doubt. A friendship that starts strong feels like an exciting new connection, only this time, something turns sour.

Many friendships have their ups and downs, with expectations being met or not, and sometimes it's a case of getting into the flow of understanding how much time you have for one another at a particular stage of your life. As friends, we have to be understanding of someone else's circumstances—like when you want to see them every night of the week but the selfish woman has gone and gotten a new job or boyfriend who is taking up all her time! How dare she?! These forks in the road happen in all friendships and yet are easily navigated through honest and kind communication if you're in a healthy space too. The truly toxic ones, however, are never as straightforward as this. Nor are the issues caused by circumstances and changes in life—they will feel consistently shit no matter what is going on because generally that person might just *be* a bit shit.

In my experience, the telltale signs of a friendship that is turning bad are often quite subtle. For me, one was feeling I was in a very unhealthy trap of constant comparison. It's very normal to compare yourself to your peers and while we all have the odd day of feeling like we're falling behind compared to others, a more constant nagging, negative feeling of comparison could be a sign that someone is making comments to make you feel this way. As I said, this can be very subtle, which makes it very hard to pinpoint what is actually happening, beyond just the feeling of discomfort you're experiencing.

Here's an example. I once met up with a friend after I had fake tanned; she commented on it straightaway, finishing with, "Hell, I would never fake tan, I just go so brown naturally." It was such a small thing, but when these sorts of subtly undermining comments come thick and fast, they build up and make you really doubt yourself—but only in comparison to them and their choices. They are making you feel this way and building on your doubt!

The trickiest thing with this is that the comments are usually such small things that you can easily brush them aside as you being petty or oversensitive. But if this feeling is cropping up week after week, day after day, then you're not. In this particular friendship, I didn't really speak about it to anyone for a while. It was my boyfriend at the time who pointed it out when he said to me, "Liz, whenever you go and spend time with her, you come home and you worry and talk about things I have never known you to really care about before." Lightbulb moment! I *didn't* care about this stuff (fake tan all you like, ladies)—what was bothering me was this person making me doubt my own taste/opinions/work ... the list went on. And all through very subtle put-downs and comments, which were then accumulating to something much bigger. I still felt like this person was a good friend to me, who I didn't want to lose, though of course eventually the friendship did end—and I have never looked back.

"Be vulnerable and notice the effect it has."

Incidentally, this person had many other friendship fallouts. I was aware of them at the time and thought it was just bad luck or other people's wrongdoings, as she was a good friend as far as I was concerned! But of course as time went on it became quite clear that *she* was the common denominator in all of these friendship breakups and would continue to be long after our friendship had run its course.

Ultimately, this girl made me feel small and not good enough, which can of course also happen as a result of far less subtle behavior: being deliberately excluded, being made to feel you're being spoken about behind your back, being left wondering what you've done wrong with no one offering an explanation. These situations and feelings are always caused by someone who is keeping the upper hand, wanting to maintain a queen bee position—it's all shit and, quite frankly, a form of bullying. So if you read this and thought of someone in your life who is ticking these boxes—get rid. You're better off without them and, importantly, the way you are being made to feel is absolutely not a reflection of you. It's them.

Once we have had those experiences, it can be hard not to carry over fears and doubts into new and healthy friendships. With social media being at the forefront of our lives, the feeling of missing out or being left out is easier to come by than ever before.

Let's say someone has texted you back in a way that's a bit blunt. Yes, they are probably just busy, but if you're having a bad week where you feel insecure and low, it can be hard to take this at face value. Instead, we interpret it as so much more: they are cross with me; I have annoyed them; they don't like me. I have finally found a friendship group and I have RUINED it and will never find another one again ...

Then you might go on Instagram: they didn't like my photo. They put a photo of a coffee on their stories; they're having drink with someone but the last time I asked them for coffee they said they were busy but they clearly have time for someone else because THEY HATE ME.

You've gone from one to a hundred in under five minutes and your friend is just having a busy day and loves you as much as she always has.

This leads me back to my main point—be vulnerable and notice the effects it has. I find I can become more sensitive to things when I have been vulnerable, as when you have given more of yourself you have more to lose. You really have to roll with these punches, use your rational mind as much as you can and put a stop to habits like looking online for evidence that confirms your fake narrative (because you will always find something and make it fit when you're feeling this way).

If you find yourself in a situation like this, here's an idea: write two lists, respectively titled "Thoughts" and "Facts." So a "Fact" is: "She didn't text back but did post on Instagram." That's it. Everything else that is pointing you to a conclusion that this person is cross with you or, even worse, doesn't want to be your friend, are just thoughts not supported by facts. Write them down, then cross them all out and try to let that symbolize you removing them from your mind too. If the feeling is still nagging, tackle it with more vulnerability and communicate. Just a simple "How is your day?" or even,

"I am struggling today, I seem to be a lot more anxious than usual." You're not blaming your friend or trying to make them feel bad but you are sending out a very small SOS and I promise you a good friend will always respond with kindness to that, and all your worries will melt away.

Let me end on the moments in those well-established friendships that bring you even closer together. You've found them, worked through any of your insecurities, and kept them in your close circle, but there are still some dramatic moments to come. Even Lindsey and I have had our ups and downs. Like the time Lindsey blocked the toilet in our hotel room in LA. This is a story that has stayed close to my chest until now. After realizing her mistake in the morning, she chose to leave the situation for a qualified member of housekeeping to deal with while we were out in the day. On returning to the room later, we realized that we had not been so lucky and the situation was even worse than when we left. At that point, Lindsey decided to take matters into her own hands, quite literally. Armed with nothing more than a ziplock bag from the airport security, she delved into the depths to try to dislodge the issue. At this point I was already beside myself with laughter over the whole ordeal, which was only made worse when she exclaimed, "Oh no ... there was a hole in the bag."

Half an hour later, housekeeping arrived with a plunger and we were still both crying with laughter.

Lindsey on **Friendships**

I don't quite know where I would be in my life without the love of my friends. The friends that make me laugh until I cry, the friends who hold my hair back when I've drunk too much, the friends I call in the middle of a panic attack, the friends I cry on when my heart feels like it won't ever be fixed again. To all of you, thank you, and I hope you know just how much I love you back.

We will experience so many different kinds of friendships throughout our lives. Some will be beautiful and some will be damaging, as we move through the stages of our lives, picking up our entourage as we go, from school to college, to university and to work—or at least, that was my path.

I didn't find any of my friends for life at school. They came much later for me, at university. I was always a bit of an outcast growing up. A proper tomboy, with teeth too big for my mouth. I wanted to be popular, to have friends to make plans with, but for some reason, this kid wasn't very readily accepted into many friendship groups. I had a couple of friends who I spent time with at school but never really outside of school. I did have some wonderful neighborhood friends, my next-door neighbors. A few girls with whom I made amazing childhood memories, and have watched them all grow up, have children, and get married.

As it goes for so many of us during our growing-up years, I was quite badly bullied at high school. It came in many forms and I suppose that made me an undesirable friend with the popular kids. From time to time, the popular girls would invite me to a party or social thing but I would be the token friend who would get picked on. It was so shit. There were a couple of girls who, now and again, would stick up for me when I couldn't do it myself and for that I will always be thankful. Spending time alone gave me a lot of opportunity to reflect on the type of friend I wanted to be to other people. Having experienced the loneliness of not having very many friends during this time has shaped the loyalty and fierceness I put into my friendships today.

My mom has also shaped the way I treat my friends and the adoration I have for all of them. Mom would always have her girls round for food and wine when I was growing up and I envied that so much. I love those women, the women my mom calls her friends. I used to want to stay up late and join in with them but when it got to bedtime they used to say, "Right sex, wrong age!" and it still makes me laugh today because that will always be the way—since there's 30 years between us all I will never get to close that gap.

My longest-standing friendship is now 33 years old. We have our moms to thank for throwing us together because they are best friends, too. We went to different high schools and universities but came together at the same college. Our moms taught us what it is to give love, loyalty, and strength in a friendship. We've survived more battles in our lives together than I can count—including but not limited to: treatment of STDs (plural) and picking up the pieces after many a broken heart. This woman even stood by me when I ditched her for a period of time in favor of my new boyfriend. Of course, I returned to her with my tail between my legs when things went belly up and she, thankfully, welcomed me back with open arms. She's the very best woman. I'd be totally lost without her. And I thank my lucky stars for her and her curly hair every day.

Talking of ditching your pals for your new partner—don't. In friendships, we want to see our friends thrive, be in love, be happy. It's normal for our friends to drop off a little bit for a short period of time when they begin a new relationship; it's all the sex! It takes up so much time! (And dealing with the cystitis!) But it's not OK to completely prioritize a new partner; you must also make time for your friends, keep in touch, check in, make some plans. Those friends will always be there, your partner may not. Nurture the relationships you already have.

Although we hope our best buddies will always be there, throughout our lives, most of us will also experience friendships that mean so much but that may only serve us for a shorter period. The kind that fizzle out, where we fall out of step on account of differing lifestyles, children, work, many other things. And this is so normal. These people come in and out of our lives for good times and good reasons. Don't try to pick this apart more than is necessary—I promise you, you haven't done anything wrong if you find yourself with a dwindling friendship on your hands, so please don't look for blame, it's likely no one's fault.

I have so many fond memories of spending important time in my life with lots of different people over the years, from falling half in love with my physio educator when I was on placement at a hospital during my training and becoming really good friends, to meeting people on the other side of the world when exploring Australia as a whippersnapper and going through so much personal growth during our time there. These people are really important to me but that doesn't mean they are in my life every day.

They say you can count your true friends on one hand, and for me I feel that is true. That's the core collective of people who know you inside out/upside down and love you despite your flaws. That's not to say we don't also have a wider circle of people we love and want to make time for. This is also true for me.

As someone who is surrounded by wonderfully talented, kind, and supportive women in her friends, I have always struggled to understand how other women don't want or need that in their lives. Each to their own, of course; you might prefer male friends, you might be the type of woman who prefers her own company. But more often than not, it's because something is a little awry. This doesn't make you a bad person, though. Something my mom told me, that has served me well this far, is this: "Women who do not have friends, cannot *be* friends." If you don't have friends, female friends in particular, then how would you know how to check in on people, to be kind, to be supportive, to raise people up?

I have learned this the hard way. I have put my love out there for people who were simply unable to accept it and they absolutely couldn't return it. That's all OK, it's life and sometimes it takes a little while to figure out why it's not working. Believe me when I say that in this scenario, it is not you—the person trying to make the friendship work. Pull yourself away and protect yourself.

Friendships are built on love, trust, and mutual effort. MUTUAL EFFORT. Read that again. I've had some friendships that have been incredibly one-sided and it's disheartening to say the least. I couldn't understand why people wouldn't put in the effort that I did. It's true that some people "just aren't built that way" and we mustn't put pressure on everyone else to behave as we do (by we, I mean givers!). However, at the same time, someone who just isn't making an effort isn't worth your knocked confidence, your canceled plans, your utter frustration and, actually, sadness, sometimes. You can lead a horse to water but you can't make it have a drink with you.

Getting over a friendship that's broken down can take some time; it's different from a romantic breakup but, hell, it hurts in its own way. Friendship breakups are fucking hard. People don't just drop off the face of the earth when you wish they would—not that I wish them harm. Maybe they could drop off the face of the earth into a big pillow and start a new fluffy life down there away from us? Sometimes we can't just wash our hands of that person who has turned out not to be a great friend and be cool to move on—sometimes they are entwined in an existing friendship group so it can be tough to navigate.

One of the things that goes hand-in-hand with solid friendships is the ability to provide "tough love". When you can see a close friend in a sticky situation, whether that's romantically, work, or something else, you are often able to offer them advice from your outside perspective, enabling you to give it to them straight when they need it most. I tend to be the giver in this department as I have a knack for sussing out where my friends are up to, when they aren't happy and what it is that's causing the unhappiness. It can be tricky to manage but as long as they know it's coming from a place of love—because you want the best for them and not "you're trying to take away my fun" or "you're not happy for me" then you stand a good chance of helping them muddle through these bits. What's a friendship without a little turbulence now and again?!

"Sometimes you have to step out of your own perspective to be able to see what is good for another person."

HELPING FRIENDS WITH DIFFICULT DECISIONS: HOW TO OFFER ADVICE

One of the aspects we find so vital in our friendship is the way we can both help one another through a difficult decision without telling the other person what to do. It can be hard to sit back and watch someone you love make decisions you don't feel are good for them, but finding the right way to express that can be even harder! Giving advice is a delicate skill at times. You don't ever want to overinfluence someone or make them feel like they're making the wrong decisions when making mistakes is a really important part of life! Over the years, we have helped each other through so many big life decisions and we want to share a recent one where Lindsey made the decision to leave London and settle down in the suburbs.

Lindsey:

I made the move from London to the countryside in June 2019, after five wonderful years of big-city living. It was a move I was ready for, one I felt I craved. I got there and settled right into it. After all, I was only one hour outside of London, one hour away from my best friends, one hour away from most of my work commitments.

As the months rolled on, though, that "one hour" started to feel like three. Unreliable trains, sometimes a three-hour rail replacement service on a BUS, the last train leaving London at 23.30 ... I let these things take away my spontaneity—the option to stay late and go for drinks, to pop into London, to stay over at Lizzy's on a whim. I had this feeling that I "must get home." As a result, a feeling of isolation started to creep in and it was scaring me. Like my youth was flashing before my eyes. A baby was in my plan (yet more isolation on the horizon) and I started to feel like I couldn't breathe.

Lizzy is the most pragmatic and logical of people; she has a way of helping me to focus on exactly what it is I feel and showing me what actions I need to take to fix it. (Though she always says, "If only this was true for myself!")

After some tears, some wine, and Lizzy taking on various devil's advocate roles, many of which provoked strong emotions, I arrived at the conclusion that I either needed to be back in London or I needed to see the one-hour travel time for what it was: just one hour. So we came to our conclusion—I would spend more time in London, stay with Lizzy more, and go to London at the weekends sometimes, so my trips there weren't all centered around rushing from meeting to meeting for work.

Soon after this meltdown, we went into lockdown as a result of the Covid-19 pandemic. I now had a new plan and told Lizzy I wanted to get a puppy. A mere two weeks after I had cried about feeling isolated. I could feel her tear her hair out from five hours away where she was in her respective lockdown. Impulsive is an understatement when it comes to me and I couldn't be more thankful that Lizzy is able to cut through my garbage to make me realize that my ideas are mostly quite wild.

Lizzy:

I think one of the main things any friendship needs is an understanding that no matter how close you might be, you're both on a different life path. With or without an age gap, you're likely to want different things at different points in your life. And sometimes you have to step out of your own perspective to be able to see what is good for another person.

When Lindsey moved out of London, I was obviously devastated. She went from being ten minutes down the road to an hour away; it was a huge lifestyle change for us both in our friendship. But I have watched her make it work, watched her make a happy home, balancing a quieter pace of life in the countryside with nipping into London however many times a week is needed. I have known how tiring it's been, how much planning it takes—and how often those trains cancel is honestly criminal! And I always reminded myself that just because I am still happy living in London and don't want to slow down, that doesn't mean it's the same for anyone else. So when Lindsey came to me to say she was feeling isolated and restless, it took all the will in the world not to just make her move in with me there and then and never let her leave! Because, selfishly, that is what I want. The closer the better, as far as I am concerned— OF COURSE this will make her happier, because it's what makes me happy!

> *"Being part of the decision process together is where we balance one another out so well."*

Well, you will all be pleased to hear, I refrained from that advice. I wasn't totally surprised when Lindsey brought this up with me. She wears her heart on her sleeve so I can often sense something is awry before she is ready to put it into words, and I know to just wait for her to come to me (average waiting time is about ten minutes). So when she did express these feelings, my first instinct would be her last one: do not make any quick decisions, all the options are in front of you, take your time to consider them all.

Feeling isolated and restless are two things that go greatly against Lindsey's character and, while the idea of her moving back to London had merits (including my own selfish ones), I knew she was more likely to make a rash decision when those feelings of discomfort were motivating her. Your gut feeling is often right, we all know this, but it doesn't mean you have to act on it instantly. It shows up to teach you something and then your friends are the people who can help to articulate it and bring the mind into the decision-making process too.

I am so proud of her, because whatever decision she may make in the future, she has lived there for a year now—that is a lifetime in Lindsey years. The puppy being the perfect example of her taking her time with a decision! She now has a gorgeous little dog that she thought about getting for almost six months, after weighing up every other part of her life beyond the pandemic. My initial concerns around this were based on her tying herself down even more, at a time when her wings were feeling clipped anyway! We spoke about it from every angle; I offered up every scenario of how she would navigate life with a dog and she had an answer ready for everything.

Ultimately, we will both support whatever decision the other makes. But being part of the decision process together is where we balance one another out so well. We each know our choices are our own to make, and that we will be there through it all—Lindsey could move back to London and back out again six months later and I would still help with every move (though maybe with a bit more tutting during the third one!). A gut feeling doesn't go away when you talk about it but it can be rationalized and turned into a plan—a plan that spreads out over weeks in my pragmatic case, or a few hours in Lindsey's impulsive one! There isn't a right or wrong, but we counterbalance each other perfectly.

◆

This scenario I am about to discuss is one I think that lots of friendships have navigated and it takes patience to do so. Something that Lindsey normally has very little of, except when it comes to her friendships, when she has it in abundance. And that is the moment you know a relationship isn't right for your best friend.

I was in a relationship that was fine—happy (most of the time), fun, exciting at the beginning. With the wonderful gift of hindsight, I can now clearly see the moment some cracks started to appear but at the time, my head was somewhat buried in the sand of just wanting things to be OK, to not really have to deal with what was glaring me in the face if I had really looked. It was one of those funny gut moments you try to push to one side, which of course only come back harder and harder. And Lindsey was having those gut feelings with me, and for me, at the same time. It wasn't a case requiring an intervention, of, "This man is hurting you and so I need to make you realize how much happier you would be without him," but more that I was denying the fact that I wasn't getting what I wanted and deserved out of something, which I think is way more delicate to address.

We were in a taxi in Copenhagen when it first came up; Lindsey said something along the lines of, "Sometimes it feels like you're keeping the seat warm for the perfect person he is looking for, without realizing it's you." I remember feeling really annoyed and defensive but hiding it, as deep down I knew she had just put into words what I already knew, in the way only a best friend can. Lindsey managed to navigate this with me in a way that didn't end in an "I told you so" gloat, but instead with complete understanding of how I had ended up there, before I even really understood it myself.

I have a tendency to overthink so much that any gut feeling gets drowned out by the power of the mind. Lindsey never lets her gut feelings be forgotten and that difference in our personalities is essential in these moments, as I needed someone to speak to my own gut feelings and bring them back to the surface again.

Lindsey:

These moments, the ones where you know something isn't right in your best friend's relationship, are some of the most delicate within friendships and, like Lizzy said, we will all go through them, whether you're the one in the thick of the relationship and you can't see the wood for the trees, or the concerned pal on the outside with a clear view of the whole forest. The closeness that Lizzy and I share means I feel what she feels and often cry if she cries (not all the time, though, I'm not a wet wipe), usually when she's at her wits' end with the situation and I'm at my wits' end with seeing her so hurt.

Her relationship started off in the most serendipitous way, a way I was so thankful to the universe for. The stars had aligned for Lizzy and it was so bloody good to see her excited and happy, and falling in love. Lots of relationships start this way—it's aptly termed "the honeymoon period" and Lizzy had a good solid one.

The relationship was long distance, which is always tricky. It started to become clear that Lizzy was the driving force in the relationship, the one sacrificing her time, blocking out her weekends (much to my dismay, but of course I remained quiet about my selfish thoughts!). I think one of the turning points for me was when she said, "If you don't mind, I want to keep the next two weekends free as I'm not sure when he will want to see me and I want to be ready to go when he says he can." My gut kicked in.

It's so incredibly difficult to watch someone you love get deeper into something you know isn't making them happy. Lizzy is a strong and extremely independent woman and the fact that she was willing to place her life on hold to fit around him did not sit right with me. I tried to guide her to think about how much she was giving up and suggested she try to ask him to share the responsibility. She was too worried about pushing him away, though when she said that out loud, her own doubt started to set in.

Over time, I picked up on further sacrifices that Lizzy was making—the one-sided kind that would be met with his enthusiasm and love-bombing to make her feel reassured that this was how a relationship was meant to be. More turning points arose when Lizzy became anxious, basing her reassurance on how far in the future a plan would be made for them to see each other. I was at a point where I could see a painful end a mile off—the pattern of hurt, anxiety, the constant tests we set out for men in our lives (even though they don't know they are being tested) only for them to fail and disappoint us. My ability to have so much perspective on what Lizzy was going through made it easy for me to understand where she was at and how she was feeling so I could raise her up and let her know that none of this was her own issue, but his. I understood completely that she had to handle it in the way she felt was right. She came to see that she was absolutely better off out of that relationship. It didn't take her too long to find herself again.

QUESTIONS AND ANSWERS: FRIENDSHIP

You go to talk to your friends about most of your issues, but who do you go to talk to when the issue is with them? Well, the answer is US. We are your friends via the words on this page; look no further.

How do I deal with a betrayal in a friendship?

Lizzy: I think mine and Lindsey's answers may differ on this because I tend to be much more of a soft touch and make excuses for people for too long. I do have a threshold somewhere but in some relationships in my life, it still remains to be seen. I have, thankfully, never been majorly betrayed by a friend. I can't imagine how painful it would be because the trust you build in friendships is such a special type of bond and love. I would say the best thing you can do is to decide if you can trust them again. A friendship without full trust is always going to be stunted, which in some cases is totally OK. Not all friendships involve sharing the intimate details of your life—some can just be with a person who is great company over a wine twice a year. But a betrayal suggests a certain level of closeness to begin with, so it may well be a case of deciding if you can relegate the friendship to a more distant realm while you rebuild your trust, or if it's too far gone. And that will come down entirely to the specifics of the betrayal and your own threshold with something like this. One thing I would say is friendships do come and go, and that is a healthy and normal part of life. So don't force something to work if it no longer serves you.

Lindsey: Hell. I don't know if I've got anything diplomatic to say here, as Lizzy has rightly called … Once you've crossed me, betrayed me, hurt me—or someone close to me—there is absolutely no way back in. It depends on the kind of person you are but, for me, loyalty is at the forefront of all of my friendships and once that's been broken I really couldn't see past it. I would have to, and always have in the past, remove them from my life.

What makes a good friend?

Lizzy: Back to the basics here! I think it comes down to one big aspect, which is being generous. Be generous with your time, with your love, with your advice, with your energy—all of those things that the right friend will give back to you, to make the friendship grow into something beautiful! This translates into practical things such as always being present when someone needs you, giving up your time to listen, and lend advice. It means making an effort to make someone feel included in your life, sharing the day to day, which in time builds an intimacy as you learn more and more about each other's lives. Also, taking the time to have shared experiences—at school and university this is done for you as you are living a shared experience; as an adult it takes a little more effort.

Lindsey: There are so many delicate qualities that go into making a good friend. One of the main things I've learned is to accept people without too much judgment; instead, you offer support, or practical advice if that is what they need. Love, trust, and support are imperative to building a lasting friendship and I wouldn't be anywhere in my friendships without loyalty, too. Friendships thrive off these things and these relationships will be some of the longest standing you ever have, so we must take care of them.

How can I build a beautiful friendship and take care of it too?

Lizzy: Maybe let's talk about what not to do. We have all had a friendship that feels weighed down by pressure and extreme expectations. Friendships need work, love, and nurturing—but they don't need to feel high maintenance. Like I have said, you will likely have lots of friendships that operate at different levels—a small handful of close friends (maybe even only one person!) who you speak to every day; some people you check in with once a week and some you don't see for months and months on end but just pick up where you left off when you do. It's always important to be understanding that people can't consistently give 100 percent, and if you are putting pressure on someone to do that, they're actually less likely to do so because the expectation feels too much. So make sure you are compassionate always and let a friendship grow at its own pace. Even Linds and I didn't go straight to being extremely close; it grew over the years, partly as our personal circumstances changed to bring us closer together. I also have friends who I see very intensely for a while as we live close by and then we naturally drift slightly when that changes. There are no hard feelings or fallouts, and if we were geographically close by again, we would pick up our old routines. Both building and looking after your friendship needs patience, kindness, and a lightness. Friendships aren't meant to feel heavy. Sure, they can't always be plain sailing, but they're not meant to feel like a weight in your life!

Lindsey: Years! These relationships develop over time and need lots of love and nurturing. As Lizzy has said, our friendship grew as we moved through life and blossomed when Lizzy moved to London and from that point we really were inseparable (still are, global pandemic excluded). Our lives were mirrored but just a few years apart and so we bonded over shared, and difficult, experiences, mainly in matters of the heart. I couldn't put my finger on what the main ingredients are but I know that without tough love, kindness, and acceptance, while also being so happy for the other when great things happen in our lives, we wouldn't be where we are now. Things change constantly within friendships—such as one person moving cities, starting families, work commitments. Sometimes your lives might not feel as in-step as they once were but this doesn't mean that things have to change. Instead, you pour more into it and make more considered decisions about the time you spend together.

How do I get my friends to recognize my achievements?

Lizzy: I think it's all too easy to respond to this with, "Well, they should if they're a good friend!"—that was my first reaction! But then I stepped back and thought about it and maybe there is more to it than that. If a friend is constantly neglectful to the point that you feel unsupported then it would be time to review that friendship. But if your friend is a really, really good one but not being as responsive as you would like about your recent work promotion, for example, maybe there's a case for dealing with that with a generous hand. Generally, people are selfish. If you don't work together, your friend naturally isn't going to be as engaged with your own work life—they have their own to tend to! And they could easily not have understood the significance of something to you. The best thing to do would be to tell him/her how much of a big deal it was to you but without saying anything like "and you made me feel like it wasn't." You would hope that your friend would then respond accordingly and give you the recognition you were craving from a person you care about so much. And the whole situation will be dealt with without any finger pointing! It would only need to be handled with a harder conversation if this was an ongoing thing, in which case you may need to sit down and explain kindly that you feel like some of your own life milestones are going unnoticed.

Lindsey: See my answer to betrayal on page 51 … ! If your friend isn't supporting you, cheering you on, and raising you up, then honestly, get the hell out of that friendship. While I understand that we aren't all built in the same way, these are the very basic ingredients to a healthy friendship. Friends shouldn't have to be told when to say "well done" or that they're proud of you, but if they don't say anything and you're hurt by that, this shows the friendships means a lot to you, so if you feel you'd like to talk it over, bring it up, because if you don't you could be left wondering what went wrong. Follow Lizzy's advice on this regarding diplomacy.

Will "friend with benefits" ruin the friendship?

Lindsey: I have had a few good friendships with men that have resulted in friends with benefits. I actually, shockingly, managed to navigate most of them really well because the friendship was strong enough. I know that this isn't widely believed to be possible, or a good idea. I suppose it's down to what you wish the outcome to be; I only ever wanted a friend and sex so it worked well for me. I was around 19 or 20 years old at the time so I think my attitude was completely different. I'm not sure how I would navigate that in my thirties with starting families and settling down on the brain. In fact, we all know I absolutely could not navigate that!

Lizzy: Oh gosh, I so wish I could say that I didn't think it did change anything but I think it does. I think the chances of falling in love with a friend are just too damn likely, especially if you have some sort of sexual attraction, and when you fall in love you naturally lose the easy breezy-ness of the friendship. Maybe it doesn't need to be thought of as ruining something because it could develop into something even more incredible but I feel it's naive to think the friendship will remain the same.

"Sometimes your lives might not feel as in-step as they once were but this doesn't mean that things have to change. Instead, you pour more into it."

CHAPTER 2

Heartbreak

We have both had our fair share of heartbreak over the years, in every form: we have been dumped, been the dumper, been messed about, been sent mixed messages, felt love fade in a loving relationship, questioned whether to stay, asked ourselves and each other the almost impossible question of "but is the grass greener?". We both stand by the belief that *nothing* can affect your day-to-day life like love and heartbreak. We are both quite emotional little souls and can be lifted up to lofty heights while in the throes of a good and loving relationship, but also find ourselves shuffling around rock bottom when that all goes to shit. Heartbreak can feel like such a lonely part of life but, believe us when we say, we've been there. All you have to do is turn on the radio to realize how universal the pain of heartbreak is; there's a good reason why so many songs have been written about how fucking awful it is!

The positive to take from this is that it will be OK. The girl you see in the bar looking carefree and laughing with friends? She's probably been heartbroken and is doing great now. The happy couple on a Sunday morning on the coffee run? Both have likely experienced heartbreak and then rediscovered happiness all over again. The man peacefully reading in a park on a summer's day, content to sit alone in silence, may well have had a heartbreak that once made even that simple activity seem impossible. It comes to us all and it gets better for us all.

> *"I adapted like a social shapeshifter to please everyone but myself because, in essence, it was easier."*

We should start this chapter by saying that at the time of writing this, we were both experiencing varying degrees of utter fucking heartbreak hotel. Lindsey a bump in an otherwise steady road, Lizzy the more floor-to-ceiling heartbreak. Some of this chapter was actually written during a trip to LA that we both so desperately needed as a result of said heartbreak. Although we realize that wherever you are, heartbreak still hurts just as much. Maybe lying in the sunshine, listening to a sad playlist takes the edge off slightly, but there's really no escape from salty tears and gut-wrenching sickness. Sorry.

Both of us have experienced heartbreak in such dramatic ways prior to this current heartbreak, too, so that's been a barrel of laughs, as you can imagine. But it means we are here to help you! Get comfy, write all over this chapter if you need to, fold down the pages (even though Lizzy hates it when Lindsey does that—especially to books she's lent to Lindsey), and keep these pages close because you absolutely aren't on your own in this and we promise that this will get easier. There are just a few things you need to get through first ...

Lindsey on Heartbreak

The thing about heartbreak is that, no matter who you are, universally we experience the exact same all-consuming, mind-fucking journey through what feels like a void, a black hole, a space so large you can never ever fill it—or at least not now. Heartbreak comes in so many forms but there are two types (in a romantic sense) that I've been through: the biggest one I've ever had and the one made up of the small heartbreaking moments that chip away at our happiness, if we let them.

Let's start with my biggest heartbreak. Ultimately, the one that shaped the woman I am now, sitting here with a massive glass of orange cordial at the age of 33:

You were on your way home. Things had been strained. I was the most anxious I had ever felt. I changed into that shirt you like so much. I swiped my lips with a bright color in the hope it would hide how fraught with worry I was that you'd leave. You still left. Despite the shirt, despite the lipstick, despite me sitting at your feet with my arms draped over your knees. Well, technically I left. Down the freeway to Stockport, Greater Manchester, with nothing but a spare pair of panties and my toothbrush in my pocket and the wettest, most salty looking face you could imagine, to the arms of my mom who answered the door, handed me a stiff drink, and caught me with her free hand. Never have I been more thankful that my mom is as physically strong as she is mentally.

That relationship was six years long, taking place in an era soundtracked by Arctic Monkeys, Bloc Party, and Arcade Fire. It was my first true love, the kind you'll walk over hot coals for without hesitation. I was 22 years old and it was the biggest learning of my life. To navigate two different people, their fears, emotions, ever-changing landscapes, educations, and families is a complicated thing to figure out how to do.

What turned out to be the pivotal thing for me at this time was that I didn't know myself without him. I didn't know my limits; what I needed in a friend; how to trust myself; what kind of sex I liked—I was a chameleon. I adapted like a social shape-shifter to please everyone but myself because, in essence, it was easier than trying to think about what my true feelings or thoughts were.

Even so, the first couple of years of that relationship were such a happy time for me. The newness, the excitement, the love. Everything was a first. I felt those things not just because I gave them out but because I truly received them too. I couldn't tell you when the shift in me happened but I became completed by him and, in turn, codependent, even though I was in total and complete love with this person. How, at 22 years old, was I to know what codependency looked or felt like? The answer is, I wasn't, pal!

I have always prided myself on being the driving force that gets things done. I'm the same in romantic relationships, too—specifically when it came to locking down a secure relationship with this person. I was relentless, I know I was. What I know now is that my behavior fed, grazed, and existed on pure insecurity. I wanted so badly to see a ring on my finger, our first child on a 12-week scan. Unfortunately, he didn't want those things with me—it took six years and a truck load of anxiety to get there.

> *"Give kindness out and feel the benefit from it."*

So back to Greater Manchester, back to the nuclear family. To the house I grew up in, to my childhood bedroom still painted in "Rodeo Drive"—a strong shade of lilac completed with a silver border to, you know, break up the room.

The only life I knew was in tatters. It did not sink in. Would. Not. Sink. In. Part of me thinks I wouldn't let it. I took, not only solace in, but clung onto every letter in every word of kindness his family sent. Though this quickly became a source of more panic because if they were reaching out, a matter of hours later, then he really was done. It was over, over. I remember lying on the couch staring at the ceiling, Mom close by, doing that thing moms do when they're trying not to fuss but ultimately are causing more fuss by not fussing. The next few things that happened will be etched in my mind always.

My dad took me to a major home improvement store, to pick some paint so we could get rid of "Rodeo Drive." He said, "We're going to give you a proper space and it doesn't matter how long you stay at home." We painted and listened to the new Bombay Bicycle Club album on repeat way past midnight until there wasn't a single trace of lilac left. In its place was a more grown-up shade of gray.

Ikea came next and Dad was nothing short of amazing. I'm so lucky with my parents, so very lucky. Though I get my fiery nature from Dad and if anything was going to crack him, it would have been Ikea on a Saturday with his zombielike heartbroken daughter in tow. Guess what? I didn't even hear him utter a single profanity under his breath. We came home with some plants, sensible storage solutions, and a special closet paint so I could do away with the dark brown wood and cover it with yet another shade of gray—like my soul.

The day after I arrived home, I was due to start a new rotation at work. I was working as a physiotherapist at a hospital local to my former home with my ex-boyfriend, a good 90-minute drive from my parents' house. Junior physios working on the wards in a hospital rotate every six months around different areas of medicine. I was moving from outpatients over to a stroke ward. I knew nobody.

I have never received kindness the way I did that first day. Of course, the patients had to be my priority but I also had to own what I was going through. I asked to speak to my manager to explain the situation and from then on, she checked in with me, made sure I ate and drank plenty. She soon became a friend. The entire team knew what was going on and were all so incredibly gentle with me. Work was the best thing for me—it gave me something to get stuck into, putting other people's serious needs before mine. Give kindness out and feel the benefit from it—I stand by this as something I would advise now, too, as it helped me much more than I could have hoped.

> *"You must ask yourself if you spend more time being happy or sad."*

A physio friend of mine and her husband were heading off to New York a couple of months after the end of my relationship. She saw the destruction to my life and invited me along on the trip with her husband, another couple, and their mutual friend. She didn't even hesitate, she searched for flights to make sure I could get a similar one and that it wouldn't cost too much money and we booked it. Having that in the diary and feeling so included did wonders for me. My friend and her husband were so important in how I worked through my heartbreak. One evening, my friend's husband was working locally to where

I lived so he drove over, picked me up, and took me out for coffee and to an exhibition. I still don't have the words of gratitude for what he did.

Over the coming months, I would date, I would watch live music, I would drink heavily, I would have plenty of sex, I would dance until my shoes had to come off. I really, really lived and tried to feel absolutely everything. One of the things (with lots of hindsight here!) that got me through was to have a diary full of plans. I'm all for wallowing if you need to but I couldn't; it's like I woke up and I changed my life entirely with a determination that could only have been born from such pain. Having a perfectly woven web of the most supportive friends and family was the only thing that got me to a place of happiness and acceptance.

In many ways, I think that the biggest cliche of all, "time is the greatest healer", is also the truest. I'm almost seven years clear of that heartbreak now and it has changed over the years, evolving into manageable pieces. The pain you feel becomes less intense; the unanswered questions remain unanswered but don't haunt you in the same way anymore. That all-consuming sadness fades away. The way you move on is your business but, above all else, you must remember that your happiness is paramount. Don't let fear control your next steps toward happiness and love. I promise you that you'll be happy again, with or without a partner, and on the day you realize that, you'll probably cry in celebration, and that's OK too.

◆

Now that I've taken you through my big heartbreak, I'd like to talk about the small ones, too. The ones that creep up on you day to day, the ones that slowly grind you down over time, the ones that make you feel like you're failing at love. I'm talking about the heartbreak you can experience during a relationship that is often, and on the whole, happy. These moments come to us all. You can be in the most loving, respectful relationship and feel that you're exactly where you need to be and with the person you need to be with, yet something you didn't expect can jolt you right out of that happiness and throw everything you thought was real into question.

As someone who bends over backward to ensure her partner is happy, it couldn't be a bigger mystery to me. It literally dumbfounds me. I would say that, for all my faults, I am a very fair person when it comes to love and fallings out. As I've got older, I am absolutely the person who wants to talk things through, to understand all sides of the debate, settle things down again, kiss, and make up. What I do not do well with is being shut down by the other person. I need to resolve things to manage my anxiety. I think so many of us operate in this way too.

Sure, I've thrown a camera tripod or two across rooms in the house—who doesn't get wound up from time to time? But dealing with someone who needs a couple of days to cool off after an argument before they're ready to be calm and kind again is a rather large headfuck. When I'm not heard, or given the chance to communicate properly, I don't feel important, I don't feel respected. That's a tough pill to swallow from someone you're madly in love with. This is the type of thing that can grind us down. There's absolutely something to be said for validation here too—it's natural to want the validation of the person you love. It's always been huge for me and, as brave as I am, I really need that from my partners. I think in some way, we all do. Oh, to be aloof!

The way I got myself through these periods is to remember that while I might think that my way, the "adult" approach, is the perfect way to deal with it (it is), my partner is an entirely different person with entirely different needs. I can't put what I think is right onto them, that's not fair and it's not how it works. With time, I've learned that you can take it less personally if you give yourself a pep talk. It's not a reflection of the way they feel about you, it's just the way they need to navigate the situation and their behavior is a product of that, even though it's difficult for us to understand at the time. We've always got to remember though, when these times crop up, that mini-heartbreak moments must be in the minority in the grand scheme of the relationship. You must ask yourself if you spend more time being happy or sad.

Lizzy on **Heartbreak**

I have had my heart broken a few times in my life in different ways. From leaving a long-term relationship, which felt like a heartbreak I was somewhat in control of, to the relationships that seem to suddenly fall apart and end abruptly. Each one has had its differences but the foundations of feelings are very much the same.

I think all heartbreaks are essentially similar, which is why we can empathize so readily when someone else is going through it. (Surely we will have all listened to a song about a breakup and felt as though it was looking into our soul and must have been written specifically for us and our experiences ...) We can all recognize the moments you feel like you're free-falling away from a life you invested so much time, energy, and love into. We know the feeling of desperation where you unpack the past, the last exchange you had, your own behavior—wondering if you could have done something differently, what might that have changed. We can all find solidarity in the moments we obsess over what he/she might be doing, if they're moving on quicker, crying as much as you are, feeling *anything whatsoever*?! We have watched friends fill with hope when their phone vibrates, only to deflate when they see it isn't a message from *them*. We all know it will get better too, that the pain will be intense and you will feel so empty inside that it's very reasonable to believe you will feel that way forever, but you won't.

Heartbreak is a grief. You lose a huge part of your life and have to go about rebuilding that life without them. The key difference is that the person who is gone is alive and well, swiping right again or making eyes at someone else across a bar. The element of choice involved intensifies the pain of splitting up—their decision not to be with you makes you feel even more out of control. It feels like an injustice because there is a very practical way that the pain could be fixed (them banging down your door with flowers and apologies) and yet they are continually choosing not to do this.

> "Herein lies the crux of letting go—you cannot do it with the hope it's going to get someone back."

My experience with this is that you fast-track through the process of grief in an agonizingly intense way. It's the debilitating sadness, the bewilderment, the anger, the guilt, and the acceptance all within the space of months. But it is the fact that they are still alive and flirting with whoever they want that makes this feeling temporary in the way that getting over a death is not. You can also flirt with whoever you want and rebuild love and happiness with someone new. So it's not as permanent as someone you love dying but it is a grief and I have experienced my lowest lows when dealing with heartbreak because of how quickly I have been plunged into a world of pain. My point is that you must allow yourself to grieve and to accept what's happening. It's the very first step of letting go—that infamous and near-impossible thing we must all find a way to do.

The idea of "letting go" has been the hardest thing for me in all my heartbreaks. Unfortunately, I have to tell you that there isn't a "how to" guide on this because, believe me when I say, I would have found it and pasted it onto my bedroom walls if there was. I once had a phone call with a psychic (this is a go-to for Linds and me in hard times, it's not for everyone, but we love it) who said to me: "He will come back to you, but only when you let go." And herein lies the crux of letting go—you cannot do it with the hope it's going to get someone back. It's very true that men have a sixth sense that detects when your energy shifts away from them and they often choose that very moment to message you again. But you cannot fake this shift—well, you can fake it till you make it, but making it is the key bit. You have to find a way to let go, to remove them as a frame of reference.

This is something I am dreadful at, utterly, utterly, dreadful. And I think it makes me the best person to dish out some advice where letting go of that love is concerned because I have tried it all and it was only really time and focusing on myself that did the trick. Oh, and meeting someone new. Why does this feel like a bad thing to admit? I feel like I should be able to pick up the pieces by myself and move on without the help of holding on to someone else between the sheets. I am not scared of being on my own but still it's always been the presence of another man that has truly kicked out the last one. For me, discovering a new person shines an even brighter light on what was wrong in the previous relationship. All the things your friends were telling you about them, all their shortcomings you've been reminding yourself of in order to get over them, suddenly become as clear as day when you throw yourself into the honeymoon period with someone new. Of course, many people will reach this lightbulb moment without a new love interest at the top of their chat list and I wish I were one of them. But whichever camp you fall into, there are definitely some things you can do (or avoid doing) to help stop your ex playing on repeat in your head.

1 Don't friggin' message them, especially if you've been dumped

Just don't do it. Not speaking will create distance; distance creates space for you and your happiness in a way that isn't linked to them. And if they are messaging you and it's not a stepping-stone to getting back together or working through the problem, then stop it. Block them, tell them to leave you alone, do whatever you need to do. But don't accept bread crumbs from someone in this moment as it will just prolong your pain and get you stuck in a cycle of being given hope, only to feel abandoned again. Breaking contact is really important for you to find space to heal from it all—but hell, I know how hard it is to do. I know how much you will want to speak to them but if you are both committing to moving on, then not much can come from a conversation.

Of course, there are times when you do need to come back together to have a big chat. But if you're doing that, don't chase the dream of "closure." From my own experiences, closure is something very elusive that has only ever finally come to me when enough time has passed and I am no longer agonizing over another person's thoughts and actions and finally focusing on my own again. Any big conversations that are had post-breakup need to be as focused as they can be. You will go into the conversation with a list of things to discuss; the other person will without a doubt say something that you will ruminate over for days and then you'll tell yourself you need *another* conversation to clear that bit up. This can go on for infinity! You have to be very strong in saying what you need to say, asking what you need to ask, and then leaving it there. Don't drag out your own pain and remember that "closure" will elude you for as long as you're looking for the other person to hand it to you.

> *"This road will not be a straight one— but the twists and turns will become less frequent."*

When you have been dumped, it's also very normal to hold onto the hope that they will message you. For me, I have to fake it till I make it. My motivation at first for not messaging will be that they need to feel my absence if they're going to want me back! And I can hold my ground with that as my goal—getting them to reach out by being the one who doesn't do it first. It's not particularly healthy but as the weeks of not speaking tick by, I do find that I move into a new post-breakup stage that isn't so focused on when I am going to hear from them. It's inevitable that you'll find yourself thinking, "When will they message me?!" But it's one to try to move away from. The more time you spend focusing on their actions, which you cannot control at all, the less energy you give to your own.

2 Find a way to fill the free time you now have with things you love

New hobbies, reading books, watching TV, drinking wine (in moderation, too much makes the first step harder to stick to)—embrace whatever it is you love and makes you feel even a little spark of joy within this misery.

3 Accept it's going to take time

This is very important. You won't wake up one morning and leap out of bed suddenly unable to even remember what their surname was. Instead, you will have a day where it gets to 11 a.m. and you realize you are only just thinking of them. You will have a night out where you have fun—and I mean proper, proper fun. You will have an evening in at home alone that doesn't involve a lot of sobbing and Instagram-stalking. Yes, you will take some steps back—this road will not be a straight one—but the twists and turns will become less frequent and more like a gradual bend as opposed to a hairpin turn.

> *"When you are looking for something online with a narrative in your head already, you will find it."*

4 Be really honest with yourself about the barriers you are building to avoid getting hurt again

It's perfectly normal to feel scared of getting close to someone again after a big heartbreak but don't allow that to prolong your pain. Don't say to yourself, "I am not over my ex, so I can't meet someone else," when really it's that you are too scared to be vulnerable with someone again. Own that reality and take your ex out of that equation so you can really start to move forward with your own intentions.

Periods of heartbreak can be a really powerful time to reflect on things. You are going to be feeling very raw and have your mind racing at 100mph all day long, so do your very best to channel those thoughts. Imagine you are taking off your rose-tinted glasses as you do that too. Really consider the relationship you are healing from and allow yourself to focus on the bad bits instead of the good. There is a reason it hasn't worked out and you must be brave and face that head on. Even if you have to write a list on your phone titled something along the lines of: "20 Reasons Why [insert name here] Is a Total Jerk Who Won't Make Me Happy and Who Doesn't Deserve Me and This Is Why I Am Moving On" that you return to throughout the day to remind yourself of it all, then do it (see page 89—we've even made you a template!).

5 Step away from social media

You are only prodding the bruise every time you have a little stalk of what they're up to. When you are looking for something online with a narrative in your head already, you will find it. Let's say we see a photo of them having a coffee in a spot you used to go to together. Where will your mind go? Mine would do something like: "He's there with another girl, it's a date, he's dating already—oh no oh no oh no." That has just taken time out of your day you could have put to something (anything!) else and has allowed your mind to spiral down so many tunnels you might not see the light at the end of it for the rest of the day!

"I have no doubt in my mind that you will be OK."

You have to build up some self-discipline here. It's SO hard to resist that multicolored circle around their Instagram profile photo. And so easy to convince yourself that within that Instagram story is the piece of the puzzle you are missing: the new girlfriend they got a week after you broke up, sobbing over how much they miss you. Both seem very unlikely—it's probably a photo of a coffee, a blue sky, a meme. Something that won't help you in any way to see but will just feed a cycle of checking their socials in the hope of clarity that you will not find there. Not speaking to them is half the battle nowadays; the full battle is stepping back from any reminders of them so you can really move on. If you have to block them to do this, then that is what you do. It's not a petty move if it's what you need in your healing. Out of sight, out of mind really does work after a while.

◆

I started writing this less than two months after my most recent breakup, in a moment when I was finally, after weeks of unrelenting sadness, finding moments of happiness and joy in my life again. I was at the point where the road is getting straighter and I could definitely see the horizon. And now, over a year on, I am revisiting this chapter to say with conviction: I promise it will get better, I promise you will get through this. I promise there is a better love out there than the one you have just lost, I promise you will open your heart again even if right now it feels like it's still in a thousand pieces. I promise you will wake up one morning and they won't be the first thing you think of. I promise you will be able to return to the places that are filled with memories you had together and it won't feel like you've stepped on an emotional land mine.

The lessons you learn from heartbreak are such a gift—a cruel one but a gift nonetheless. Every relationship I have had, and every man I have loved, has been informed by these experiences. Knowing what I do and don't want, knowing what my personal red flags are (though I am likely to ignore them anyway—that is a lesson I have learned too), knowing what I value and what niggles I can live with. It's a journey and if you happen to be at the point of your journey where you are experiencing the pain I have just shared here, then I am truly sorry, but I have no doubt in my mind that you will be OK.

If you've read that last paragraph and are still feeling like, "No, I will not be OK. I am losing my mind, I am never going to get back to myself," then, especially for you, here is a list of things I have done while heartbroken, just so you don't feel so alone:

❡ Cried publicly and loudly in not one but TWO different central London sandwich stores. I can't look at a chicken and avocado wrap without feeling some level of PTSD now.

❡ Made Lindsey sit down with me and rate the likelihood of various outcomes: "Will he message me?" "If so, WHEN will he message me?" "Will he be sleeping with someone else right this very second?" And so on and so forth. Sometimes I even tried to make her put money on what she thought would happen, to really test her judgment. (She hasn't yet ever agreed to part with money for this, which is probably for the best. Although, on the other hand, she does normally predict it really well so she ought to put her money where her mouth is.)

❡ Googled "celebrity couples who have broken up and got back together" to get a sense of the time scale of these breakups. I did take some comfort in knowing their experiences would have had parallels to mine, no matter how famous they were.

"The saying 'time heals all wounds' couldn't be more fitting for a broken heart, so just keep putting one foot in front of the other."

❡ Cried so much that one of my eyes swelled up and I couldn't fully open it for an entire morning. This actually happened in an airport and I then sat slumped against a pillar aggressively sobbing down the phone to my mom.

❡ The usual unrelenting social media stalk, in which no stone is left unturned. You reading this might not stop you from doing it but just know, no human in the history of the world EVER felt better for having done this. Yet we all do it. It's the painful reality of feeling there is so much information readily available that might answer the burning questions we have. When really, we just make whatever we see fit into the narrative we are trying to create. And ALSO, if you do see something you want to see and it peps you up a bit, it's not mature communication at all. If they have something to say they should be able to reach out and say it—anything less is a black mark against their name.

❡ Written down so many thoughts I could actually start a local library full of my own little sad handwritten books. This isn't a bad thing; I recommend you write it out over and over—journaling is a powerful tool throughout this. A good way I was taught to start doing this was to write one A4 side every morning. It's a lot of space to fill but it teaches you how to write in a stream of consciousness.

¶ Sat and stared at a messaging service to see when they pop up as "online." I am not sure what I thought that would bring to me; it didn't help with anything. Please don't waste your time with this one.

¶ Moved house, three times. An expensive and stressful solution but actually, for me, this one helped. The sense of a fresh start is more exciting in a new environment and it's always given me a sense of control in my life again. Even if moving house with a broken heart is a true test of strength, it's doable.

> "There's really no escape from salty tears and gut-wrenching sickness. Sorry."

There are so many more nuances to heartbreak than just being dumped, too. The ones that aren't getting over someone after they leave, or you make the difficult decision to—what about the ones that can come up while you're in a relationship, whatever stage that relationship may be at? The stable and established one that hits a big bump in the road, the one that suddenly falters after an exciting beginning, the agony of an on-and-off one that leaves you reeling. It's easy to see heartbreak only as a reaction to the end of something, which then kick-starts the process of grief, but there can be so much more to it than that.

There are so many different versions of this scenario; whether it's someone stringing you along, someone telling you they need a "break," which leaves you confused, someone who isn't ready for the relationship you want but still doesn't want to lose you, someone who begins to withdraw after months of something feeling steady. These are situations we can all find ourselves in for months (even years!) with a person.

The cycle of hope and disappointment, hope and disappointment

This can be entirely heartbreaking because it can lead to you staying in a situation you believe you can fix and then, as the constant problems recur, it often feels like a reflection of you, of something you are failing at. It makes the attachment so strong it can feel impossible to break, no matter how many days you spend feeling utterly lost and devastated by the situation. Those days of devastation can be alleviated by the other person, by their reassurance or attention, making you feel like you aren't failing after all! And before you know it you can find yourself in something codependent.

The fact of the matter is, until you want to give someone up, you rarely will and this can be a heartbreaking position to be stuck in, or to watch someone go through. An analogy my counselor once gave me is imagining that you're the guy in the movie *127 Hours*. Your arm is stuck in a rock—only this time you're stuck between an emotional rock and a hard place. Until it gets so painful that you have to cut off your "arm," severing that attachment and that part of yourself, you will find a way to stay in the relationship. People find their way back to each other countless times until one of them is strong enough to say no and shut that door. You can sit with your friend and tell them to leave someone who is making them unhappy until you are blue in the face, knowing this will plunge them into a deep pool of heartbreak that, in the long run, is still less painful than the long shallow one they are currently wading through. But until a person is ready to go, they will not.

On the flip side, it can be really heartbreaking to be the person who is doubting the relationship, to be the one cutting off someone else's arm (OK, let's ditch this graphic analogy now!). Perhaps this is due to a big argument in which hurtful things were said that cut deeper than you thought possible, and the argument feels like one you might not get back from. Or maybe it's the unrelenting dread of being in the "beginning of the end" phase that we all pretend isn't actually that, until it's impossible to ignore what's right in front of you. It could just be a tricky patch that you will both navigate and then come out the other end stronger, but looking at a person you were once so sure of and feeling a pang of doubt is heartbreaking in itself.

Being dumped, being the dumper, being the person with the doubts that can sometimes feel so intense it feels like a daily betrayal—all these experiences have been some of the hardest things I have ever experienced. But whatever side you find yourself on, it will be OK. The clarity you are searching for will come to you; the pain you want to leave will start to fade. The saying "time heals all wounds" couldn't be more fitting for a broken heart, so just keep putting one foot in front of the other.

HEARTBREAK

Here are some thoughts you will have during this time of unbelievable pain, when you feel desperately out of control and will gladly grasp onto any form of control that you can find to prove that you are not mad. You might feel you are alone but you certainly are not—we have all been there.

1 I wonder what X is doing now?

2 Will they realize they've made a mistake? Definitely. How could they not?

3 Maybe this is the kick in the ass they needed? The old saying, "You don't know what you've got till it's gone" ... Surely that's true ...

4 Will I ever sleep again?

5 We just need some time apart to realize we are meant to be.

6 Damn I want to text them. Even just an emoji would be OK, right?

7 Oh hell, who will their next partner be?

8 ARE THEY HAVING SEX AGAIN?

9 Am I hungry? No, it's just wind.

10 I'll text and check in with their mom, just to be kind, I loved her too!

THE PHONE LIST REMINDER

Here is a template for a list you can keep on your phone for whenever you need to remind yourself of why you're on this horrible journey, and that it will get better. Let us help you take off those rose-tinted glasses and then stamp on them and smash them into smithereens so you don't ever put them on again.

> *"The clarity you are searching for will come to you; the pain you want to leave will start to fade."*

The aim is to have a long list (15-ish entries) to look at and remind you why your life is going to thrive without them. You can make it as specific as you need. And you must have it on your phone so you can consult it as often as you need to, and also add to it as you go. You can even copy it out a few times if you need to, to make it stronger in your mind. This is a good way to attempt to control your thoughts. Consider getting it printed on T-shirts for your friends to wear. Maybe some wallpaper for a feature wall? Go as far as you need to.

This is a list to remind you why your relationship with
[...... NAME HERE ......] didn't work out and why you are
moving on

Try to include:

❡ AT LEAST three things that they didn't give you. Did they
communicate enough? Were they selfish at times? Did they
always prioritize you?

❡ Something they did that always wound you up! There will be
something there and it can be as specific as you like.

❡ Let's have some times in there when they didn't appreciate
what you did for them. It's important to know there is someone
out there who will not only appreciate those things but also give
you the same back.

❡ What are your nonnegotiable traits in a partner? This is good
to have going forward and it's unlikely that the relationship that
didn't work out will have ticked them all.

❡ Your next goals in life and how you are going to achieve them
alone—which you are 1,000,000 percent capable of doing!

❡ And finally ... let's try to get the ICK in here too. See next page
for more details.

THE ICK

(Purposefully written in capitals due to its sheer power)

The Ick is going to return later in the book, so if you're not familiar with it, best get to know it now. You have likely experienced it yourself. "The Ick" is the term used to describe a feeling that fully turns you off. From looking at the bend in someone's fingernail for too long to watching someone you like dance. It is something that makes you want to close your legs and wrap them into a pretzel shape. It makes your butt hole clench. It makes your teeth set on edge.

Many of us come across this feeling during our dating careers. It can be anything and, one day, it just gets you and there's no going back. It's been known to be a really helpful tool when you aren't sure how to end something. The Ick spurs you on and enables you to leave without sadness. Long live the Ick. It's very important to know that this isn't a list of things you shouldn't do. Everyone can do these things and not give the Ick but the wrong person doing them at the wrong time has induced the Ick ...

1   Watching as a man I really fancied closed his eyes softly before kissing me—but way too early pre kiss. I swear I've never made my excuses more quickly. Goodbye.

2   Someone saying that they have "a funny tummy."

3   I had a boyfriend at uni who once got into bed, lay on his side looking at me, patted the bed, and asked me to get in. I wanted to run the other way. I didn't want him or his penis anywhere near me. Typing this out makes my skin want to leave my body.

4   When someone bends down to pick something up and you can see the top of their butt crack.

5   When someone smells something bad and does that hand waft motion in front of their face.

6   One time, a boy I was with tripped over his words in a group conversation and then made the "blurblrblerghblrrr" noise with his tongue to correct himself. But he just did it for a bit too long and it was honestly excruciating.

7   When you're ignoring someone who is doing something and they want your attention and you are determined not to look so they start doing it more and more enthusiastically and you can just see it unfolding in your peripheral vision.

THE BREAK UP FLOW CHART

You can barely remember to eat. Getting out of bed is a chore. You didn't know you could cry this much. Every waking thought revolves around THEM! Here is a little flow chart to get you through, to get you back to functioning day to day and to remind you there is a light at the end of the tunnel.

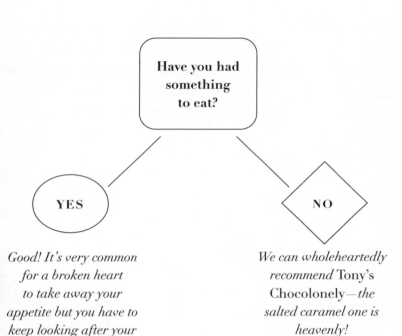

Have you had something to eat?

YES

Good! It's very common for a broken heart to take away your appetite but you have to keep looking after your body just as much as your mind!

NO

We can wholeheartedly recommend Tony's Chocolonely—*the salted caramel one is heavenly!*

"There are so many more nuances to heartbreak than just being dumped."

How many times
have you watched
"Buffy the Vampire
Slayer"?

ONCE OR
MORE

NEVER

*Once more,
with feeling!
(Buffy reference there,
but you'll know that!)*

*We grant you
permission to put this
book down and head
right toward the TV.
Seven glorious seasons
await you. And Buffy
is also the heartbreak
inspiration we all need!*

*"Take off those
rose-tinted glasses
and then stamp
on them."*

When was the last time you spoke to your best friend?

JUST NOW

Call them again and insist on making plans that revolve around a sensible amount of alcohol.

I'M NOT SURE, I DON'T WANT TO BUG THEM

Call them and ask for a distraction. And if you are worried you're putting too much on them, then explain that and let them know you won't be offended if they ever need a day off from it. Chances are they will always be happy to talk and help you through this bit, so make sure you lean on them and ask for help when you need it.

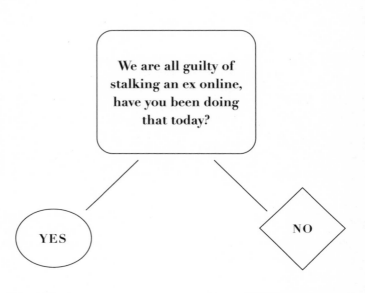

We are all guilty of stalking an ex online, have you been doing that today?

YES

NO

Go and admit this to a friend so they can appropriately tell you off for it and remind you of all the reasons not to.

Congrats! Have a glass of wine to celebrate and leave your phone in another room. You know whatever is on their social page will be boring anyway.

"Please don't waste your time with this one."

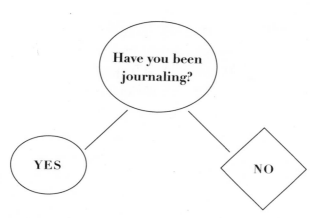

Have you been journaling?

YES

NO

Good! I promise that one day, many years from now, you will be moving house and clearing through your cupboards. You will find this notebook and read one page filled with all that sadness and you will not believe how far you have come! And the person trapped in those pages will feel like someone from another lifetime. This sadness you feel right now will not stay with you forever.

Come on, give it a go. Walk to your local stationery store and treat yourself to a nice new notebook. Go for something chic and simple. Get yourself a pen that feels lovely to write with too — Lindsey and I are big fans of the perfect pen (it can't be too thin and scratchy but also not too soft). Head home, make a brew and just write whatever comes into your head. You can draw, you can scribble, you can write lists. This notebook is yours, for your eyes only.

Have you given
enough thought to what
YOU are doing/feeling/
wanting today?

YES,
FINALLY
I FEEL IN CONTROL
AGAIN

EVERY
WAKING THOUGHT
IS OF MY EX

You have come so far!

*Keep that focus on the
most important thing
right now: you.*

*"This sadness you feel
right now will not stay
with you forever."*

Are you spending enough time fantasizing about all the men/women you are yet to meet and fall wildly in love with?! Who, by the way, will be better than your ex.

ERM, YES, AND I AM TEXTING THEM

NO, THERE IS NO ONE ELSE FOR ME

You are through the darkest days! All the excitement is at your fingertips and you are ready to grab it. There is so much around the corner that will be amazing!

Simply not true. You need to go for a walk with some great music and daydream like mad. Have all the fantasies about who you might meet. Where you might go. All the opportunities coming your way! That beginning bit of a relationship where it just feels like heaven on earth? You are going to have that again with someone incredible!

CHAPTER 3

Grief

This has been the hardest chapter to write for us both. While we've been writing this book, Lizzy has passed a significant grief anniversary and Lindsey has said goodbye to her beloved Nana. It's given us the insight to write about grief both from the perspective of years on from an experience and also in the immediate aftermath of an event that shakes your existence. The podcast episode we made about grief received by far the most feedback and we were flooded with messages about your own experiences. The bottom line for so many of you was this: thank you so much for talking about it, I feel less alone hearing someone else's experiences. Because grief is nothing if not lonely.

We all wade through it in our own ways, at our own pace, and at times even the most robust support system of family and friends can't fill the aching loneliness. We hope, once again, that sharing what we have been through might help that in some way, however small. Even if only to remind you that it's OK to feel alone and lost. You aren't doing anything wrong; you're doing your best and, under the circumstances, that is remarkable.

"Eleven years on, I am still digesting. This is why grief is a lifelong journey."

Lizzy on Grief

I don't really know how to talk about grief. I hope that is a very relatable line, because who really does? It is a sudden abyss in your life; someone goes from your present to the past and all we can do is reminisce and hold on to the memories and love while trying to move forward. To try to come to terms with what it means to know you'll never, ever see that person again. One moment they are there, breathing (however labored), and then the next they are not—and with that, everything you knew of that person is gone and they are relegated to the past tense. How can anyone comprehend something so huge? I am here to tell you that I cannot and it's OK if you can't either.

Yet grief is a huge part of my life and identity in so many ways. I have lost four family members. First, my auntie Susan when I was aged eight. My grandma when I was 11. My auntie Jenny when I was 14. And my dad when I was 17. I am 28 as I write this and it's a strange thing to say how relieved I feel to have gone an entire decade without any more death in my life. I can say with confidence that life goes on—maybe on a new trajectory, as something so huge reshapes so much of you, but it continues forward nonetheless and it continues to have the moments of happiness and lightness you knew before. This is what I want to share: the painful story of my grief and the joyful moments that have followed, despite the odds seeming to stack against this at times.

The first death I experienced that I have clear memories of was my grandma when I was 11. She had cancer and I can vivdly remember when my mom explained it was terminal and what terminal meant. We were driving around a traffic circle and it was the first time I had ever tried to comprehend the fact that death was imminent for someone I loved. At age 11, grief and death still feel like very grown-up, Mom and Dad problems. And I suppose your parents hope to control the way you are exposed to these things at such a young age. They have to deal with difficult questions—will you let your child see someone who is hours away from death, will they attend the funeral? These were all decisions taken out of my hands.

> *"It is a sudden abyss in life; someone goes from your present to the past."*

When my grandma died, I was staying at my cousin's house. I woke up and walked downstairs to see Dad stood at the bottom. I instantly knew she had died and that was why Dad was there, and the fact it was Dad, who was strength and protection, meant it was all OK. I never considered that this was a man who had just lost his mother. At that age, as far as I was concerned, Mom and Dad didn't have an existence outside of being my mom and dad. The only way I can really remember this grief manifesting was in a relatively short-lived period of being scared of sleepovers, so clearly some sort of separation anxiety from Mom and Dad. There was more than one instance of Mom having to come get me from a friend's house in the hours of the night as I'd got so worked up and begged that someone call Mom.

Thankfully, that fear of sleepovers went away after a while.

◆

I spent many weeks in the various school vacations at my auntie Jenny's over the years. She lived with her husband Luigi (who was 25 years older than her). Jenny and I used to write each other letters and cards starting "Dear Best Friend" when I was at home in Leeds. Every summer at least, I would have one week at theirs. Jenny was the coolest aunt ever, in a way that would have stretched far beyond my 14-year-old opinion if she was still alive now. She was so stylish, so charismatic. Just the other day, Mom and I were speaking about her and one of her lifelong friends. I asked Mom where Jenny had met this friend, to which Mom said, "On the tube." Nothing could be more Jenny, starting a long-standing friendship on the train line. Jenny charmed people everywhere she went, with a husky southern accent, the longest legs you ever saw, and a uniform-like wardrobe perfected to a T.

Jenny died very suddenly when I was 14 after having a brain hemorrhage. Her death was the first time I remember understanding the adults around me as actual people, beyond their relation to me. Seeing Mom upset made her more human and less just "Mom," seeing Luigi's (Jenny's husband) grief made me understand him more and seeing Dad jump into action and support everyone made him seem even more superhuman than I already considered him.

The days immediately following Jenny's brain hemorrhage were full of the grisly decisions about keeping her on life support, donating organs, and when to give up on hope. Thankfully, I was too young to be instrumental in those decisions but I remember the days well and watching the way adults somehow managed to function and be rational and measured in these extreme moments.

> *"I feel less alone hearing someone else's experiences. Because grief is nothing if not lonely."*

I miss Jenny so much as an adult; out of everyone in my family, I am most like her. Just last weekend, Mom came to visit me in London and berated me for not having properly dusted anywhere, saying, "You are just like Jenny." Sometimes I walk through my house barefoot and notice the soles of my feet are a little dirty and it transports me back to their house that was full of stuff and never that clean. I love stuff, hate cleaning, and actually love living in a state of semichaos most of the time. I have the same hands as Jenny and the same moles (identically placed) on my arms. When we go to Italy to visit Luigi, he often remarks that I am the only stylish person to walk in the door since Jenny last did (he's biased because I now wear very, very similar things to Jenny and wish we had kept her wardrobe as we are the same clothes and shoe size too). Physically, Jenny lives on in me and I couldn't feel luckier for that.

◆

As I have mentioned, Dad was the strongest man I have ever known, and will ever know. I don't know how to put into words what it feels like to miss someone this deeply, other than that it's a feeling that physically hurts my heart. If I think about how much I wish I could pick up the phone to call him this very second (especially to tell him I am writing a book, he would be so proud), it feels as though someone is grabbing my heart and squeezing it. It has never stopped feeling very unfair that I can't do that and there is not a single thing I wouldn't give up to be able to speak to him again.

Dad had been unwell for a lot of my life, surviving cancer numerous times before it finally, somehow, managed to beat him. I say "somehow" because to me, Dad was invincible. I had watched him fight off cancer five times before, so even during the two weeks leading up to his death, I had no comprehension that he might not get better—because it was Dad, and yes, it's cancer, but that isn't a big deal with him. It may as well be the common cold (which, in true man form, he would tend to be more dramatic about).

This perfectly demonstrates the naivete of losing a parent, especially at a younger age. They are the person who is there to protect you and so the idea that that person cannot protect themselves against something is totally unfathomable. So even though Dad hadn't got out of bed in over a week (unheard of for him, even after huge operations he was fighting fit again so quickly), even though he had lost a lot of weight and was starting to turn a funny shade of gray and not quite look the way he normally did, I still thought he was going to get better next week and be watching the next Manchester United soccer match by the weekend. So when Mom sat me down to explain that he wasn't going to get out of bed again and the doctors thought it would maybe be a month at the longest (he died within the week), it was entirely impossible for me to digest. I can offer no advice on how to deal with news like this and, like I say, I haven't had to do it in my adult life where my understanding and perception of a situation wouldn't be shrouded in this teenage innocence. All I can say is, eleven years on, I am still digesting. And this is why grief is a lifelong journey.

I don't know the person I would be had I not experienced this grief at a young age. I have no idea what parts of me have been shaped, or even defined, by that loss. Perhaps this is a common question for anyone who experiences grief as a child or teenager, or when you are still moving through your formative years. I am an old soul, but was I before this loss? Or did the loss make me that way? As I said earlier, there is nothing I wouldn't give up for the chance to see my dad again, to hear his voice, smell his smell, hold his hands, hear his breathing. But also, I am happy in my life and it's impossible for me to know how different it would have been without living with this grief.

> *"We all wade through it in our own ways, at our own pace, and at times even the most robust support system can't fill the aching loneliness."*

◆

The year 2020 started off with the tenth anniversary of Dad's death. This one loomed over me like no other had before. An entire decade, more than a third of my entire life, had now been lived without the presence of someone I hoped would see me through many, many more years than he was able to. This anniversary was a very thought-provoking one for me and made me reflect a lot on the significance of having lost my dad at the age of 17. At 27, I looked back on the last decade and realized it was the one where more had changed than in any other period of time in my life: one long-term relationship from beginning to end, my fair share of heartbreak, living in three cities, starting a career that didn't even exist the last time I spoke to my dad. Coming into my own independence in a way I never imagined I would reach, with success I never envisioned either.

I think your twenties are the decade that sees the most changes for the majority of people and dealing with grief alongside that has left a big hole with lots of unanswered questions. What would Dad think of my work? What would he say if he knew I was writing a book (a lifelong goal of his!)? Would I be able to speak to him about men? How would he have consoled me through the heartbreaks that have felt like such a huge part of my twenties? Would he think I am funny? Would we still have the same interests? Would he love the music I have grown to love, all through the influences of what he made me listen to? (Believe me, it took years of being forced to listen to Bob Dylan before I actually started to like it.) What would he say if I told him how much rent I pay? What would he think of the way I dress? What would he say about all the piercings I have in my ears now? I could go on and on. But the bottom line is, I don't know the answers to these questions. I can give a very educated guess to many of them but I am a different person at 28 to who I was at 17, and he didn't get the chance to see me grow from a teenager to a woman. Nothing better describes grief than the all-consuming feeling of injustice that I have in the middle of my heart as I write that sentence.

> *"11 years on, the grief is a stream that trickles along beside me and less of a tidal wave that flattens me."*

It's simply not fair to live a life with these unanswered questions and yet so many of us do. And I think that is because you can live your life striving toward what you want the answers to be. Would he be proud of me? Unbelievably so. Would he support my mistakes? Yes, as he made many of his own. Would he laugh at my jokes? Of course, anyone with a good sense of humor should! He would adore the woman I have become and I wouldn't be that woman without the years I spent with him—but also the years I have spent without him.

Of course, a life with grief can be filled with happiness too. It's a massive part of me but I would describe myself as a happy person despite that. The biggest thing I am trying to learn as an adult is how that grief manifests in who I am now and in my behavior. In the immediate years after Dad died, I didn't want to speak about it with anyone, I was a closed book on the topic. It was only when the relationship I was in at the time faltered in some way that my mom gently pushed me into therapy.

Many years and two different therapists later, however, and I still haven't spent a huge amount of time opening up about this loss in my life. I am not sure I will ever not bristle a little when someone tries to lead me down that road or respond without having the biggest lump in my throat. I can truly say the sadness I feel when I think of Dad is unlike any other and feels as though it is burning through me. But one thing I have been working on recently is understanding how that loss, at that age, affects my relationships and responses nowadays.

I think therapists are sometimes disparaged for relating everything you say back to your childhood but we learn so much about relationships from what we witness in our parents, relationship as a child, and from any traumatic experiences in your early life. I have learned that the fact I didn't understand how imminent Dad's death was has likely now left me with some abandonment worries. When Mom had to explain just how serious things were, my body would have reacted with "fight or flight." Someone was about to leave, forever. I couldn't stop it; I had to just prepare (incidentally, I have huge gaps in my memory from this time to being about 18 years old and can remember barely anything of the days leading up to and months following Dad dying, which affirms the instinctive coping mechanism that will have kicked in then and continues to shield me in later years). As an adult, when I feel someone I love withdraw, my reaction is nothing short of hysterical at times. My therapist has explained this could be that memory of the moment I was told Dad was dying playing out again. And even if in these situations it isn't a death, there isn't even an inevitable outcome beyond my control, the hysteria still kicks in as my body relives a past trauma.

"The death of a loved one is something we carry with us always."

Now, this isn't going to be the same for anyone who has lost a parent and I assure you, I can become hysterical about something that isn't bringing up any childhood trauma. But as I get older, I am feeling braver and more prepared to uncover these potential links between that huge event and the woman I am today. And, more importantly, I realize now that ignoring this and not taking responsibility to develop and understand this side of myself could be more damaging in the future.

Now, 11 years on, for the most part grief is just a stream that trickles along beside me and less of a tidal wave that flattens me. There are some bad times, like when I lost the watch I always wore that belonged to Dad. I had broken up with my boyfriend the night before and was flying home from Amsterdam in a total state of shock. I sobbed my way through the airport and realized too late that I had lost my watch at security. I had never experienced self-loathing like that before and I hope I never have to regret anything as much again as I regret failing to really check the tray at security.

But for the most part, I am so happy. I live with Dad in my thoughts and heart every day and his memory really hasn't faded in the many years since I got to see him last, which is perhaps the thing we fear most when we are grieving—beginning to forget the person we loved.

LINDSEY ON **Grief**

While we can all understand grief to some degree, it will almost certainly manifest itself in a multitude of ways from person to person. The death of a loved one is something we carry with us always, as the grief, pain, and hole they have left behind changes, eases, and shifts into more manageable feelings on a day-to-day level over time. I can't tell you how long that'll take—it's your journey, your love, and your hole to fill. But with time, things will feel less intense. That's not to say you should feel guilty as you feel less sad either, we just carry the people we've lost with us in different ways as we go through life without them.

Sidney Holland. That's my grandad. My dad's dad. A man with the kindest face, the man from whom my height comes (I'm almost six foot!). As a child, I was never away from my grandparents' house. At every opportunity I got, I'd be gunning for a sleepover. Grandad was into horse racing; he was a betting man in every sense. And from what I can remember, he was pretty good at it too. I would go around their house collecting those (what I thought were special) mini light blue pens that hailed only from the bookies. Grandad was a quiet man and in some ways I think he struggled to interact with the grandkids who were hell bent on playing Power Rangers all over the living room, leaping from couch to pouf as he tried to watch the racing or the news. Can you blame him?!

My adoration for Grandad grew as I got older. After I moved away to university at 18 years old, I was able to share parts of my life with him as an adult trying to find her way, sometimes asking him for advice or receiving his unsolicited advice! His main annoyance with me, he told me when we sat together, was that I moved too fast through life, I never stopped to look after myself. He told me to slow down over and over again. He was right. He would tell me that he thought I was a movie star and he would beg me to get married in Stockport so that he could be there.

> "That feeling, that collapsing inside, is something we can never prepare for."

Grandad lived until he was 93 years old. He was ready to "go" before that. He was ready the day they took my nana into a dementia nursing home. Watching him miss her is still one of the most painful things I have ever witnessed. Strong in spirit, pigheaded in decision-making, and resistant to any help—that was my grandad.

Grandad had a fall at home, sustained some serious injuries, and landed himself in hospital. The bad turned worse. I raced from London to Stockport and stayed a while to visit him daily, sit with him. My heart broke, I knew it wasn't good. My experience in working with the elderly gave me information I wished I didn't understand. I read his notes.

I had a trip to America planned with Lizzy and at this time the doctors were saying he was stable, he wasn't getting any worse. I would be gone for one week. I wanted to cancel but my family insisted I go as there was nothing much I could do. I gave him a kiss, told him I loved him, and that I'd kill him myself if he didn't get better by the time I came home. He laughed. We held hands as I left until I couldn't reach him anymore. I turned back to look at him as I got to the door and he was still looking, smiling, and I knew. I knew that would be the last time I would see my grandad.

I checked in every day during my trip to the words "no change" echoing back at me down the phone. I knew that meant things weren't good. Grandad had a tattoo on his forearm of a pinup-esque woman in a leopard-print dress holding a sign above her head that said "India." I got that same tattoo during my time in America. He'd have killed me.

The day I landed back in London, Mom phoned me to say it wasn't good. My next thought was to book a train to head back home but something stopped me. I couldn't bear to see Grandad in any other way than I did last time—he was still him, still smiling, and we had had our goodbye.

The next morning, my phone rang at 7 a.m. It was Mom and all she could manage was, "He's gone," and we both hung up. That feeling, that collapsing inside, is something we can never prepare for.

For the next few months, I coasted through life, feeling like I was living inside a quiet box. Not much made me happy. I thought about him constantly. I couldn't bear anyone showing me kindness for fear of breaking down. That's always the way, isn't it? When you feel at your most hurt and most vulnerable and someone shows you kindness or love, you lose it.

The hole he left behind in my life can never be filled. As the months and now two years have passed, the way that I adored him has come to outweigh the intensity of the hurt that was once there.

> *"Although I have moments that reduce me to tears, on the whole, I pull on the very best memories."*

I think there's a common misconception that when we lose a grandparent, it's sad but it's OK, it's not like it was a parent. I say bullshit to that. It all depends on how big a part of your life they have been. My grandparents have had a huge bearing on my life, on the person I am and that love is family love, regardless of what name the relative goes by.

◆

During the period of time that it's taken to write this book, I lost my nana, Edna. The other half to Sidney. When I said at the beginning of this chapter that grief manifests itself in different ways, I honestly wasn't prepared for how losing my nana would hit me in such a different way to when I lost my grandad. The love you share with your grandparents is so precious, so particular. Losing them both has taught me that I felt such different strains of love for each of them. Both wholly overwhelming.

My nana was the person I was desperate to spend my weekends with, the person who let me raid her closet and flounce around in her own mother's fur coats that were left to her. Her cookie jar was something to behold and the lemon cake, wow, the lemon cake she used to make— I've still never had one as good to this very day. After bath time, she would let me use her Royal Jelly body cream. I still love that smell. She was there for my school plays and my dance classes, and she spoiled me rotten. My nana was one of the most active people I knew, she never sat still! She walked everywhere and was determined never to let her age stop her. She was always in the backyard, tending to the flowers of which she was so proud, or sunning herself— she would go the most beautiful shade of tan which highlighted lots of white scars on her arms from all the knocks and bangs she sustained from being so clumsy, just like me. Nana loved to dance and she loved to sing, she was full of joy but also had the best feisty temper on her. There are so many similarities between Nana and I, right down to our matching curved little fingers on both hands, that look like they could have been broken at some point.

For the last four years of her life, Nana suffered from Alzheimer's, a form of dementia that essentially robs people of themselves, letting them fade into people neither they nor we can recognize. It is a heartbreaking situation, knowing that person is physically with us, but not mentally.

Every time I went back up north I would visit Nana in her nursing home as a priority. She was high-spirited, hilariously witty and cheeky, and would brighten my day no end. I have to admit, through tears, that as her disease progressed, the anxiety that visiting her caused me ultimately stopped me from visiting her so often. The day she couldn't remember who I was was too much for me to manage.

My nana was my dad's mom, so I had to talk to him about why I didn't know if I could carry on visiting. Of course, he totally understood. To my nana, my dad walked on water—he was the absolute golden boy, which really made me, Mom, and my brother laugh when she was alive. When she passed away, though, I found it incredibly difficult to watch my dad grieve. Knowing that someone is in so much pain and being unable to stop that pain is a terrible feeling. I can't imagine losing either parent and to see Dad lose both broke my heart.

It's been six months since she passed away. While I felt an intense, sharp bout of grief at the beginning, I seem to have taken so much comfort in believing that she and Grandad are finally together again and, although I have moments that reduce me to tears (Christmas is particularly hard), on the whole, I pull on the very best memories and have so many photos of them both in my phone that I often scroll through.

"You will learn to move through life with them as part of you and your memories."

QUESTIONS AND ANSWERS: GRIEF

Grief is one of the hardest topics to talk about. Nothing feels normal in grief because your normality has just been robbed from you and navigating that will bring up all sorts of things in your mind. We recommend you voice them when you feel ready and we are here to help. But ultimately, with something as complex as grief, professional counseling can be the best way forward. Lizzy has been in counseling on and off for seven years now and can honestly vouch for how life-changing it can be. We hate the thought that *any* negative stigma can be attached to seeking help. The important thing to remember is that it's nothing to be scared of. It can be totally normal to feel that, when you sit in that room, all the barriers you have carefully put up over the years to protect yourself will come falling down and leave you in a nonfunctioning state. This will not happen. Anything your mind and body feels is too much to process it will keep subconsciously protecting you from in whatever way it can. A counselor will help you gradually peek above the tops of these barriers and—slowly and carefully—gain a better understanding of what is on the other side.

There are no "wrong" questions to ask about grief. Here are some that we have found ourselves thinking about in the past.

How long will the loss of a person hurt so intensely for?

Lindsey: This is so difficult as we will all work along our own time-line as we go through the pain. I think when we lose someone, the way in which the grieving hits us has a lot to do with the circumstances under which we lose them. With my grandad, it was unexpected and down to an accident and so I feel I grieved intensely for a longer period of time than I did when I lost my nana, which was the result of an awful degenerative disease and somewhat expected. There isn't a textbook answer here but what I do know is that it won't feel this intense forever. You will learn to move through life with them as part of you and your memories. Try to find your way back to the normal things in life to keep you moving forward. You will need time, and that time is yours to do with what you need, so if at first you need to stay in bed then that's exactly what you do. We can never foresee how it will affect us until we are in it, so you must be gentle with yourself during this time. There is no wrong way to grieve.

Lizzy: As with any sort of pain, we want an end date on it. Wouldn't it be so much more manageable if we knew when it would stop? We could endure it so much more easily that way. But of course, there is no clear answer to this. I can say from my own experience, 11 years after Dad dying, that most days I am 100 percent OK. I have periods where grief comes back to me, but for the most part, it lives with me without slowing me down. But if you've just lost someone now, hearing "11 years" isn't going to feel helpful, I understand that. So all I can say is that there will be good days, maybe even in the immediate weeks after your loss, when someone or something successfully distracts you from your sadness. And the main thing here is you must not allow guilt to follow that good moment. You don't love/ miss/care for that person any less just because you had a day where it felt easier to get out of bed, where you laughed at a joke, or sang along to an upbeat song on the radio. The person you have lost would want those good days for you more than anything and you must embrace them, and trust that, over the next few months and years, they will come with increasing frequency, until they outweigh the bad.

How do I start to rebuild my happiness after they've gone, and not feel guilty about that?

Lindsey: I promise you, it will come. For me, the happiness started to come back to me with the small things, such as wanting to spend time with my friends and making sure I did this, as afterward I would always feel so much better. I have always maintained the thought that the people we love wouldn't want us to put our lives and happiness on hold because they aren't here anymore—they would want the exact opposite of that! The guilt in this is something that might hit you out of the blue during a really happy moment. Just remember you're allowed to be happy and to carry on as normal, so try not to beat yourself up because it's all a process that you will move through in your own way and, as I mentioned before, there is absolutely no wrong way to do this.

Lizzy: Guilt is definitely one of the hardest and most complicated emotions involved in grief. Loss and grief are an inevitable part of everyone's life and it comes to people at different times—some people live with it from a young age; others live well into adulthood without it. But whatever way it comes about, no one is prepared and the foundations of your life are inevitably tilted. BUT, there will always be so many aspects of your life you remain in control of and these are what you must keep focusing on.

When someone dies, the immediate aftermath is a whirlwind of logistics and paperwork. Extended families that see each other only at funerals and weddings often bring some sort of drama, and then there is the painful part of dealing with the physical things a person leaves behind. This sweeps us all up initially, along with the focus on the funeral itself and having that big event looming over you. I would say the first step to rebuilding any happiness is to remove all expectations from yourself about how you may cope. For example, if you decide the funeral will make you feel better and give you closure but in reality the public display of grief hits you harder than you thought, you may feel like you have taken a step backward ... *You haven't.*

There are no steps backward in the process. It's going to be like a river that ebbs and flows and you have to accept that, even though it's incredibly difficult to do. Something wildly out of your control has just happened, and to go with any sort of flow means relinquishing more, at a time when you likely want to cling on to any control you feel you have left. But think of it this way: this person has gone, you couldn't stop it, but the world is still turning. You still manage to get up in a morning (even if it hurts), you still manage to eat a meal (even if it's just cereal), and maybe you managed to send one text message today. You are putting one foot in front of the other and you know in your heart that you will always manage to do that. So try to think about how strong you are already, even in these small moments, and accept that some days will be hideous but you know they will end.

In time, the good days will be here more and more often and you have to believe how much you deserve those good days—and that you deserve to be happy, even without that person here anymore. Feeling better doesn't diminish how much you cared for the person you have lost. In fact, whatever that person taught you, whatever role they had in your life, mostly set you up for those good days in one sense or another, and to rob yourself of them robs you of the legacy of the person you love too. Keep moving forward, it's going to get better.

I didn't visit my loved one before she died because I didn't want to remember her that way — is that bad? I feel guilty about it.

Lindsey: This hits home for me as I battled with this too. Ultimately, if it's what your gut told you at the time then you made the right decision. I made the same one and it proved to be the best thing for my mental health, and for my memories too. Be soft with yourself—I bet your loved one didn't want to be remembered in that way either.

Lizzy: No, this is never bad. The chances are, she wouldn't have wanted you to see her in that way either. The important memories are of times spent when someone is alive and well, not in their final days. A situation like this is a reminder of how much we should cherish those we love and give them as much time as we can, so that whenever this heart-wrenching day comes, we have so many memories to carry on with us that go way beyond the final days of care. No matter your age, seeing someone who is terminally ill is often distressing. The situation you are going through is hard enough as it is and you are allowed to set some boundaries within this process to help yourself cope as best you can.

What do I say to someone who has recently experienced a loss?

Lizzy: Accept that nothing you can say is going to make that person feel better; there is no magic answer you can give to soothe. If anything, your presence and support is the most valuable thing, which could be expressed with "I am here to talk or help with practical things at any time you need." Simply emphasize how much you mean that. In those early days of grief, the day-to-day load of life can suddenly feel like the biggest task, and so having someone to help with that can be so welcome too. Going over to clean the dishes, change the sheets ... any of those chores that just take one small load off a person's mind, when that person is at total capacity.

Lindsey: I have supported a few of my friends through grief and what I can tell you is that there is no right thing to say. Instead, I found the best way to support them was to let them talk as much or as little as they wanted, knowing I would be there day or night. I made sure they were eating properly, plied them with chocolate and, when they were ready, I organized fun things to do together. As someone who has also received love and support from my friends during grief, these things have worked for me too—the more practical approach, and just knowing that should I need anything at all, my friends would be there without question.

CHAPTER 4

Confidence

It's easy to think of confidence mainly in terms of how we look, how we feel in our own skin and our bodies, and how we want to be perceived by the world. But in reality, it's a huge topic and a theme that underpins all of these chapters in some way. Confidence is so often broken down by a bad relationship or breakup and built up again by a new love. It is nurtured in good friendships or sometimes deliberately undermined in toxic ones. It is also an integral part of what we're going to discuss in the next two chapters, *Dating* and *Sex*—as they can both make and break your confidence at times. Living our lives online, we have also experienced the many, many ways in which social media can play on your confidence too.

On the surface, we are both confident people. Sharing yourself online means you have to have some level of self-awareness. We both feel confident in our skin as adults, take the good days along with the bad, and understand it's a journey. But at the same time, we are also both anxious souls. We can worry ourselves into next week, lie awake for hours at night ruminating and doubting every aspect of life, and need regular debriefs from one another, that often start: "This might sound crazy, but what do you think about...?" Which feels like another part of the complicated ways in which confidence works (or doesn't, sometimes) for us.

The bottom line is that self-doubt—whatever shape that takes, whether it's criticizing yourself no end while you look in the mirror, doubting your decisions, questioning your position in life, or just worrying yourself into a place of inertia—comes to us all at times. Even people you look at and think, "Yep, they've got their shit together," will be having these moments too! What matters is how you learn to navigate this. To manage your expectations here, we aren't about to give you the guidebook of how to do that—we can safely say that neither of us has perfected this yet! But we will share our own experiences of the highs and lows.

Lizzy on **Confidence**

I am writing this chapter during a phase of low self-confidence. I have fallen into a cycle of making little effort most days with my appearance and I am struggling to get out of it and find the will to actually make an effort, possibly out of fear that doing so won't make my confidence grow. At least if I say I am not making an effort, it makes sense to not feel my best?!

We all go through these highs and lows of self-confidence I think, throughout all stages of life. Mine, at the moment, is linked to a lot of emotional stress, which, to be frank, just makes me look tired. It always makes me lose weight and, in turn, that makes me not eat so great in an attempt to keep some weight on, which doesn't make me feel good either. A vicious cycle that I know will fade in its own time as my mental health evens out again. I strongly believe what is going on in the inside shows out the outside too.

"Confidence is so often broken down by a bad relationship or break up and built up again by a new love. It is nurtured in good friendships."

What is especially tricky is the way the cycle feeds itself. Mentally you feel a bit bad, then it starts to show in your self-confidence, so you might feel worse and so on and so forth. And as I am in a cycle of this right now, here is what I plan to do to help myself out of it a little:

¶ Keep exercising! Even if it's once a week, moving your body makes you feel so much better anyway and starts off a positive cycle instead of the miserable one! My favorite type of exercise is a long walk, with good music in my headphones. I have never once been on a walk and come back into the house feeling worse than when I set off, even if I am soaking wet.

¶ Keep having fun. I don't restrict myself right now with much, as I think living life to the full helps straighten out my mental health a little bit and then leads me to finding more balance once I feel a little happier.

¶ Read, read, and then read some more. It's the best distraction and the best way to wind down at the end of the day.

¶ Focus on things that *aren't* about physical appearance. I think an emphasis on what's going on inside leads to feeling more invested and confident about the outside appearance, and to focus on that bit first just feeds the vicious cycle.

Like I said, confidence ebbs and flows for us all. I have had periods of feeling so confident about myself; when my body feels strong and healthy and clothes just seem to look *good* without much effort. I have felt so good in my own skin when wearing barely any makeup. I have had phases of loving my own personal style and spent every day feeling so stylish, like I am not putting a foot wrong with my sartorial choices. And this has always coincided with times when my mental health has been strong, when I feel like I have the time and energy to devote to caring about how I look.

As much as looking and feeling effortless is always my goal, I think we all know that it does take a level of effort to achieve. Invariably, the times when I genuinely don't care are when I feel worse about myself—even though not caring seems to be something we are meant to strive for. But I guess without the feelings of self-preservation and self-care, really not caring about your appearance doesn't lead to a happy outcome.

The backbone of my self-confidence comes from clothes and fashion. I am such an advocate for how great a good outfit can make you feel. I have worn jeans and a sweater that made me feel like I can conquer the world, put on dresses that made me feel brand new, and lounged at home in comfies that made me feel so content. I have also experimented with outfits where I leave the house and feel uncomfortable and not like myself all day. I've worn heels that bit too high and tottered about like Bambi and felt like an idiot and I've attempted to make something that looks great on another person work for me, with disastrous results. Personal style is a lifelong evolution with mini breakthroughs that can really keep you on the right track—realizing I suit navy blue more than black, finding the perfect pair of jeans, investing in the most perfect pair of Celine loafers that I would honestly be slightly heartbroken to lose. These are the little wins and when you strike them and leave the house in those loafers, the navy knit, and the perfect jeans, it can make you feel *so, so* good.

It's strange how it feels harder to talk about the ways in which you are confident. It's ingrained in us that it's arrogant and so it's far more endearing to others to put yourself down. Tasks like "write down three things you love about yourself" can seem impossible, and yet we could probably write a novel rivaling *War and Peace* in length about the things we don't like. But that's so unhelpful when you think about it, so I will give it a go here.

If I do say so myself, I think I'm quite funny and often laugh at my own jokes (which arguably isn't a sign of being funny but I believe I am an exception to the rule with this!). It gives me a huge amount of social confidence when it comes to meeting new people and, despite being quite introverted, I never struggle to make new friends.

> "It's so easy to forget the things about ourselves that we like."

Having good people around me gives me SO much confidence. I look at the people in my life who are so incredible and inspiring and I can't help but think I must be doing *something* right to have found myself surrounded by people like this.

I am confident in my own taste, which is quite a broad one, but in the past couple of years I really have begun to know for sure what I do and don't like. It's taken years of trial and error, but I am finally at a point where I trust my own judgment in taste.

Writing down the ways in which we feel confident is such an important practice. Even just doing that here has given me a little boost! It's so easy to forget the things about ourselves that we like and be our own worst critics, so it takes a conscious effort to turn that practice on its head and instead become our own biggest cheerleader.

> *"I am fortunate to not be too affected by these comments, even when my mental health is struggling."*

There is a specific time in my life that I look back on and think it may have been the most confident I have ever felt. It was around September–December 2018. It's hard to identify the separate elements that made me confident at that time, but let's give it a go because this demonstrates all the aspects that go into a period of self-confidence.

Firstly, I turned some sort of a corner with my personal style. It's when I found my stride with what feels most "me." Very, very simple touches like a great leather belt, some brogues, a white T-shirt collar poking out of a crew-neck cashmere knit, layered with some gold necklaces. I know how insanely specific these things are but they were hugely impactful at the time and contributed to a sense of enjoyment in getting dressed every day and just feeling great. My hair reached a length I had wanted it to get to for ages; I was getting more confident with wearing less makeup (another confidence journey in itself!). I don't mean to sound like a total idiot when I say this but, in short, I felt like my overall personal aesthetic was coming together.

I was sad for more days within this three-month period than I was happy, which also feels significant because I was finding confidence in myself in new ways despite having a hard time personally. My confidence at this time also came from work; I signed with a big agency, which felt like a huge achievement, and it goes without saying that when work involves sharing your outfits online every day, feeling good about what you're wearing really does make that easier.

The other side of that, of course, is that documenting your life online and leaving yourself open to trolling can wreak havoc with your confidence, too. It can raise new aspects of self-doubt you never had before or tear you down in the aspects of yourself where you did have confidence. It means you have an alarming number of photos of yourself to overanalyze and then an audience to do that for you too. It can all lead to strangers managing to home in on your deepest insecurities, making them feel all the more noticeable. As you try to navigate your personal style and image, linked with all those ebbs and flows of self-confidence, doing so in the public eye can make it all feel so much more intense. Here are just a handful of public comments I have been sent over the past few months about myself and my style and, believe me, these are on the milder end of the spectrum:

"Lizzy fails so badly trying to look preppy, but she only looks like a sad rich British boy in high school. She's not intellectual or interesting enough to even reinvent herself as preppy."

"The sight of those skinny little ankles poking out of half-mast pants makes me so sad. The addition of loafers/brogues makes me cringe, it's a look that is beyond ugly."

"She used to dress slutty, much closer to her true personality, but now she dresses like a granny shopping for groceries."

I am fortunate to have quite a thick skin and not be too affected by these comments, even when my mental health is struggling. I have somehow managed to internalize how I feel about myself and really only use my own opinions as a frame of reference for where my confidence is at, but no one should have to read things like this about themselves. It's human nature to be validated by the approval of others, just as it is human nature to feel insecure and damaged when we are vilified. That being said, there are times when nasty, personal comments have reduced me to tears.

The issue of trolling online is one that thankfully is being taken increasingly seriously, but there is still the constant argument that if you are sharing yourself online you are "asking for it" and opening yourself up in a way that gives people the right to criticize. This could not be further from the truth. No one, no matter what they do for a job, is "asking" to be bullied—and this is what trolling is. Just as in any office or within any work culture, no one deserves to be ridiculed in this way and made to doubt so many aspects of themselves. It is a dreadful side to the Internet that I think has the power to bring so many people's confidence crashing down around them and, in the worst cases of all, destroy someone's mental health, as we have witnessed in heartbreaking instances.

"More than ever I am questioning what I want and I feel like I am lacking direction in a way that I haven't experienced before."

Furthermore, what does it say about the confidence of those leaving these comments? Not to offer sympathy where it isn't deserved but this to me is another major symptom of how the online world has changed our confidence: the need to bring people down is bigger than ever and the ways in which we can do so anonymously makes it easier than ever, too. You can now even find communities of strangers bonded together by insulting a person they don't know. What a (quite literally) vicious cycle this creates: our own confidence is lacking and the opportunity to attempt to build it up by tearing down another person is at our fingertips. It really is the minority of people who do this but it doesn't diminish how enormous the effect can be.

◆

This phase of low confidence for me has been throughout 2020—a year in which we can all agree we had to be very kind to ourselves, and which probably contributed to the overall lack of confidence I am feeling. It's so hard to put into words but I think I just feel a little lost.

I have found being in my late twenties really strange for some reason. I am sometimes reticent to talk about age like this because I know someone in their thirties reading could find it really irritating. I don't mean I feel old at all, I feel really proud of where I am for my age. But more than ever I am questioning what I want and I feel like I am lacking direction in a way I haven't experienced before. I am not in a stable relationship right now and feel sort of ashamed to say that does make me doubt myself in some ways. Just like there is a societal pressure to get married and have children in a certain order at a certain age, there is also a more "modern" pressure to be totally OK with being single, to be able to say you're independent, and just LOVE IT 100 PERCENT OF THE TIME!

"Everyone's path is different."

Well, I don't. And as I see more friends tie the knot, get engaged or get pregnant it can be easy to feel a sense of falling behind in some way. I think so many people have similar thoughts at all stages of life and, after a year like 2020, when it's been so hard to move parts of life forward in a world that was forced to stand still, it can feel even more frustrating. But I do know I am not behind in anything. I do know everyone's path is different. I do know that the confidence of 2018 will come back under different circumstances. And I firmly believe that we need phases of low confidence as a frame of reference for the good phases too!

Lindsey on **Confidence**

People who have known me since childhood will tell you that I was the ugly duckling. One of those girls at school who was timid, bullied, and blossomed later in life. From an unsure, gangly, flat-chested teenager to someone (they say!) who would look good in a garbage bag. That's quite a nice compliment, isn't it?!

I don't think confidence is something we're born with. It's something we acquire—from our surroundings, family and friends, what people put into us, and the relationships we have. This includes the situations we have to navigate too. Good and bad.

At school, I was a pushover. I was a good girl, kept my head down, was polite, tried to fit in, was easily influenced, and had no sense of self. I became what people projected onto me. Nobody thought I was pretty, nobody thought I was worth true friendship, and absolutely nobody wanted to kiss me at the school dance. I'll tell you what though, I excelled at athletics—this gangly body was good for that! The 100-meter sprint, hurdles, and high jump were my things and I kept those safe just for me. People cheered me on at field day and that's what made me feel validated and confident in my ability. The scoreboard didn't lie and so that gave me what I needed to power through school.

There wasn't a week that went by at school that I didn't have a stomachache. Sat in the nurse's office, vying for her to ring my mom to come and collect me. I knew all the right things to say to get myself home—"I've just been sick in the bathroom, Miss." I wanted so badly to be at home, safe, where I could be myself. Bullying played a huge part in my life, thus knocking any shred of confidence I had clean out of me. Knowing what I know now about the way I'm wired up, the stomachache must have been caused by worry and anxiety. A bully pulling your skirt down in front of everyone in the lunch queue will do that to you.

When I mentioned earlier that confidence can come from what people put in, I truly believe this is true. My mom is one of the strongest people I know and she instilled a level of that in me throughout my childhood (and still does)—I had no trouble answering her back! Mom was my biggest champion in confidence, especially when she could see how much damage school life was doing to me. She was also the mom that was known for marching into school furious that I was being so badly bullied. The mom (and dad) who paid a family friend and cab driver to drop me off and pick me up from school because those bullies would try to follow me home and threaten to hurt me. If she'd have been allowed near those girls, I would have feared for them.

As a side note about my wonderful mother and an insight into where my more feisty, confident moments arise from, there was once an incident at the park when an older girl spat her drink in my face and I was drenched. The gang of them followed me home and waited outside my house shouting things at me. They nicknamed me "bullfrog" so that's what I could hear them shouting. Excellent. I got into the house quickly and, of course, Mom demanded an explanation. She saw the girls outside, got the spitting offender by the scruff of her neck, and dragged her to her parents' house to tell them what she had done. WHAT A WOMAN. My hero. They never bothered me again.

"I'm at my happiest when I'm in love and feel love reciprocated."

Once I left school, confidence started to come a little easier to me. My body had changed, I was becoming more woman and less girl. I grew into my features (teeth and ears mainly). I found my sense of style, which was basically a paired-back Sporty Spice. I was every inch the tomboy, living in soccer shirts, tracksuits, with hair done—gelled—and maybe some mascara. When the time came to go to college, I swapped out the trackie bottoms for jeans and really felt good about my body. College was an eye-opening experience for me. Boys. Boys everywhere, and boys that might want to kiss me! Hallelujah! I met my first boyfriend at college and we were together for three years. That was a huge confidence boost for me, someone on my side. I had a great group of buddies too, all mixed in with his friends. Lots of us were couples and we had lots of parties, went for sophisticated group meals, spent every Christmas Eve at the local Indian restaurant together. We had traditions! It was such a fun time in my life.

We all go through periods of time in our lives where we dislike one or more of our own physical features. I think that it's a rite of passage, a fairly normal thing to feel, to pull apart in our minds. Torture ourselves with, if you will. When I was a teenager, things seemed to be a little less complicated than they are today—hell, I didn't ever think I would write in a way that suggests I'm ancient now but here we are. WINE ANYONE? But seriously, we had the cruelty of our peers and our own minds to contend with but absolutely not a sniff of social media. And as if cruelty of bitches at school and our own mental health isn't enough to be dealing with, some bright spark launches a platform that can be incredibly dangerous for mental health, body hang-ups, and direct comparison. If I see one more face without a single pore or blemish online ... Sorcery. Must be.

Not to go on about my age, but the more I have grown in this world, the more my attitude toward myself has changed. My relationship with my body started out with unkind thoughts and words from others and then ultimately from myself—my flat chest being the main focus. I have always been and will always be too much of a wimp to have surgical augmentation so I was more on the side of chicken fillets and stuffing socks in my bra than a boob job—the kind souls at school once made up a song about me wearing socks in my bra too, that was nice. If we skip a decade or so, I like my boobs. I don't love them; I wish they were a bit bigger. But I won't ever complain about a part of my body that is allowing me to live my life again. I am healthy and I am happy.

In the same vein that my relationship with my body has developed into more of a love story over time, I am also so much more sure of myself generally, too. Life's knocks and jubilant times both affect confidence and it's important for us to take notice so we can move through it without losing sight of who we are.

Matters of the heart have always been the biggest breaker or maker of my self-confidence because I'm at my happiest when I'm in love and feel love reciprocated. It's something that's taken me a long time to identify and, now that I understand it, I'm also a bit better at looking after my self-confidence outside of a relationship. For me, being productive and organized builds my confidence, wearing my favorite socks even builds my confidence! It's important for you to recognize what that is for you. Is it love? Is it your career? Is it a skill or talent? Did your cat finally catch on to what that litter box is for? I don't care what it is as long as you can identify what makes you feel confident and keep it close.

SOME THINGS WE DO TO HELP WITH CONFIDENCE

❡ Stay the hell away from social media as soon as you notice a dip in your self-confidence. Limit your time spent scrolling. Engaging with social media affects you in ways you might not see. It can make you compare your life to the carefully curated, online-only versions of others, which can knock your confidence further. Try not to give a shit that Brenda down the road has bought a new car that's taken pride of place on her social media accounts with her sprawled on the hood, or that Jackie just got engaged and will not shut up about finding her friggin' soul mate.

❡ Pick a part of your body that you love and love it even harder. Celebrate it often and in the mirror!

❡ Put on something that you know you love, the one thing you always feel so amazing in. It might be your favorite bra, that pair of jeans that fits you in exactly all the right places, or the comfiest sweater you own.

❡ Talk to your buddies and tell them how you're feeling. Friends are our own personal cheerleaders, so use them!

❡ Write down a list of things you've achieved recently, no matter how small you may think they are. Then you can see in black and white that you're doing an amazing job of things.

❡ LIPSTICK. Underrated. I put some lipstick on and I feel more confident.

❡ Have a long shower or bath, use your best scrub, bath oils, then drench yourself in moisturizer and take some time out to get back to basics.

Lizzy on Lindsey and Confidence

Now, while confidence must come from within, there is no harm in having a little leg up here and there. Lindsey and I are poles apart in some ways and one of those ways is our areas of confidence. This goes beyond how we feel about our bodies/appearance and is more about the confidence we have in decision-making and life planning, which is where outside help can be really valuable. This is a matter of having confidence in yourself in a totally different way.

I am someone who lacks confidence in my own decisions sometimes because I don't seem to really feel a gut feeling. It's something quite elusive to me, which Lindsey possesses very intensely. I tend to sit and think and think ... and think ... and then think some more! I don't usually act for a while. I write it down. Worry a lot. Return to thinking. Write it down again, in a different notebook. Then I text Lindsey, who can give me a very quick and reasoned response.

Of course, when it's not something you're in the middle of yourself, you can have a certain clarity, but I also watch Lindsey go about her own decisions with the confidence to follow her intuition. It's not like I see her acting with reckless abandon but more like watching someone be in touch with their head, heart, and gut simultaneously and be guided by all of them. For me, my head outweighs it all and very quickly sends me down into a spiral of overthinking and hugely doubting myself. Let me elaborate with a specific example and from this hopefully you will be able to see if your inner confidence is more aligned with mine or Lindsey's.

I am going to use the age-old example of classic overthinking here: texting a boy. I could have been in a relationship with someone for months and months, know them intimately, understand on an instinctive level that one message will not send everything I know and love spiraling out of control. BUT, in that moment of needing to convey something difficult—whether it's a question I might not want the answer to and have been avoiding; a suggestion for something that could be rejected, or the classic "what are we?" that scares us all—I cannot act in a confident way at all. This is the sort of thing I will have to come to Lindsey with (probably numerous times) for her opinion. Even though I know the person on the receiving end of this message best, my confidence in my own judgment on the matter goes totally out of the window. And it leads me to the point where I don't know if I even should send the message, even when it is a decision I was once very sure on.

It starts a cycle that goes around continuously until I make my decision—hit send or delete? And Lindsey's gut feelings/decision-making helps me to come to a resolution. I don't think I have ever sent her a message asking what I should do and got an "I don't know" in response. She just always knows—and it isn't to say she is always right (I will get to this in a minute) but she always has a strong sense of how to act, which I can agree or disagree with.

One of Lindsey's less successful moments of advice came while on a trip to America. I had been agonizing over whether to ask a certain question to a certain man for a while. A few cocktails in, Lindsey's gut feelings mixed with Dutch courage came into play, and we drafted the perfect message to send. "Only something good can come from this," she reassured me. She opened my chat to check if it had been read. At that VERY moment he replied, so the message showed as having been instantly read. And while I am not one for playing games, looking like you're sat with a chat open waiting for the reply isn't ideal. We both nearly threw my phone into the pool and then almost did it again once we read the reply, which was far from what I had hoped for.

> *"You give me the gift of confidence. The strength to know that I am enough and what I do is enough, too."*

I was in bits. I am pretty sure I even sobbed through a fancy dinner we had booked and then later left my phone in an Uber and made Lindsey run barefoot down the street to catch up with it. But herein lies the crux of my confidence issues with something like this: I just want to be in control and it's when I have to relinquish that control that I feel cut adrift. Sending a message like that one means putting the ball into someone else's court and while the risk is always there that you might not hear what you hoped for, it's better to at least KNOW that rather than live under a delusion.

Lindsey has a greater "trust the process" attitude than me at times and can confidently go with the flow in a situation where I want to grip onto everything. I watch her have a confidence that things will be OK and if they're not, *she* will be OK. That's fundamentally what I lack, which is why I spend so much time thinking about the possible outcomes, thinking about how I feel, worrying myself into a frenzy—it's an attempt to predict the future, find control again, and thereby find my confidence in how to act. Linds has been a total guiding star for me in so many situations because of this fundamental difference in our personalities.

Lindsey to Lizzy on **Confidence**

Dear Lizzy,

I could count on one hand the times that you have not wanted to look in the mirror, not wanted to make an effort to make yourself feel better, and you always push through those moments and ride them out until you know you're ready to make a change, and not a moment before. Including skipping shower day—you have always hated washing at the best of times!

As a friend to me, you give me the gift of confidence. The strength to know that I am enough and what I do is enough, too. Thank you endlessly for that.

Seeing you move through life with the thickest skin of anyone I know is nothing short of an inspiration, especially when your job seems to invite the strong and sometimes negative opinion of strangers. This is where you shine, in your work, and you will not let anybody touch it or interfere with the plans you have for your future. The security you exude is catching!

You aren't just shiny in your work, though. I admire the fact that you aren't a people-pleaser. You don't need the validation of others because you know you are enough, you know that what you have to offer is the best of you and if people don't see it, or want it, then it truly is their loss. I'm getting there with this part, under your wing, in a way.

You would do anything for your friends, but when it comes to acquaintances you will cross a road or duck into the nearest store to escape a mundane "Hello, how are you? What are you doing around here?" You have been known to shush me and drag me in the opposite direction of anyone who isn't a friend because you are incredibly confident in who "your people" are.

I want you to know that for those few days where you don't feel like yourself, avoid mirrors, and skip showers, that you are loved very much, that people respect and admire you, your creative brain and the good you put into the world. Don't forget it and never change. But maybe have a shower, please.

Linds xxx

Lizzy to Lindsey on Confidence

Dear Lindsey,

You are one of the most self-assured people I know, who has that quality mixed with the perfect level of charm and humility so that it could never, ever be seen as arrogance. You make me feel safer in so many decisions because of how inspired I am watching you trust your own judgment. I can't count how many times you have said something to me in passing that has then almost become a life mantra for me to hold on to. Even when I speak to other friends (I do have some, but not many), I always find myself referring to your words and your advice and passing it on to them. You are a #influencer in more ways than one!

Your confidence in judging someone's character is honestly flawless. You can pick something out in someone straightaway when it would take me six months of saying, "I am sure they didn't mean it like that," to even begin to notice. Your intuition with things like that is incredible. That, mixed with your compassionate nature, means you just deal with relationships—friendships or romantic—with this amazing balance of boldness and softness. You speak your mind in the most nuanced way, set your boundaries in a gentle manner (and then hold them so well), and simultaneously show a kindness that lets people know they can always, always come to you. And know they will always get your honest opinion and a lot of your time.

You have a resilience that I admire so much. You just get on with things in a certain way, pull yourself out of the dark days, and make the most of every situation you are in. This is, in some ways, what I see to be the source of all your confidence. You don't wallow, you don't complain, you don't feel sorry for yourself, and you do not blame the world. You are your own woman in the most confident way, and it's nothing short of infectious.

Lizzy xxx

CHAPTER 5

Dating

Out of the two of us, Lindsey has been the most prolific dater (she really has earned the use of that word), though, unfortunately for Lizzy, most of the dating occurred when she lived in Manchester, before the friendship blossomed into what it is today. On the other hand, it is probably for the best because it's almost worrying to think what would happen if we both found ourselves single at the same time!

Dating is such a big subject that always comes up between friends. Everyone is a sucker for a dating story of any sort— the total car crashes, the love at first sight! We still hear phrases like "Tinder success story" being bandied around for those couples who met on the app (hello Lindsey and her current boyfriend!) because for some reason that feels like something where the odds are stacked against you. In some ways it is true; before dating apps, whenever you met someone there would normally be *some* common ground. It could be a mutual friend, work, even just being in the same bar you both like. With online dating, there needs to be no preestablished connection at all, no matter how tenuous. So it makes sense if it feels harder to meet the right person. But also, on the other hand, how exciting is it that you can now meet someone you would never ever have crossed paths with before?! Nowadays, the idea of meeting someone in "real life" can feel like the gold at the end of the rainbow, so maybe it would be better to shake off that idea and accept the way the world of love works nowadays. We both have friends who have met partners in a day-to-day setting and ones who met online and seen how both circumstances have led to happy and loving relationships.

"I just could not think of men in a casual way; who would be my next boyfriend?"

We want to talk about dating beyond first meeting someone though, which opens up the even broader topic of LOVE. And what a topic that is. We both go all in when we fall in love (partly why our friendship works so well, because we also give each other 110 percent) and have both been burned and rewarded for being such romantics. But whether you hold your heart back or wear it proudly on your sleeve, no one can deny that falling in love is one of the best, but also scariest, experiences you can have.

LINDSEY ON Dating

I was late to the dating game. Well, at least, the dating game had radically changed by the time I got to it at the age of 26. Enter, Tinder. At that time, it was an app for sex and sex alone, unless you specified otherwise, which in my experience would send the men I had so carefully swiped right on catapulting into the abyss, faking their own deaths to avoid anything other than a fuck. This was going to be a big leg up (over ...) back into the proverbial saddle. It's a good job I've got long legs and the determination of a thirsty camel stranded in the Sahara.

Fresh out of my aforementioned long-term relationship, I was absolutely shitting myself and excited in equal measures. Coming out of a long-term relationship left what can only be described as "a long-term relationship void" and wow, did I try to fill that. To the women who can date, have casual sex, take it for what it is, and not become surgically attached to the man, I fucking salute you. I just could not think of men in a casual way; who would be my next boyfriend? The ones that I didn't like I was able to bin off at the drop of a hat because that was within my control and also I get the Ick (see page 90) quite easily for someone who is so prone to attachment.

Welcome to Tinder

So into it we go. Tinder. At my family home post breakup, sitting on the floor of my childhood bedroom. Swipe, swipe, swipe, match, match, match, marriage, marriage, marriage. The perfect approach to online dating if you ask me ... !

The first match was a foul-mouthed, dirty-talking tall man whose first line was, "You look like the kind of girl that has a nice pussy." For fuck's sake. Talk about a baptism of fire. I went downstairs to make a cup of tea and tried not to look my parents in the eye.

Subsequently there were many matches, many chats—some taking flight, some dwindling into nothingness—along with some blockable offenses and weird-looking phalluses that I absolutely did not wish to see.

> *"This was a learning curve, but one that I would take absolutely no notice of."*

Lots of women I know cannot stand the small talk, the rigmarole of trying to impress another person with quick wit and "cool" interests. I really enjoyed this part—getting to know someone that way, the chance to show off without being physically sized up in real life. Please note that I also enjoyed it when it reached the stage of a message popping up that said, "How's your day?" Just the thought of someone thinking of me would fill me with happiness. I think it's fair to say that we all agree that I romanticize everything. EVERY. THING.

My first proper Tinder date was with nothing short of a very lovely man in Manchester. We had talked for about a week online and he asked me on a date. I was buzzing. I found him interesting, a man sure of himself without the arrogance that had been pretty evident in previous dating app matches. A gentleman, who was good at conversation and a perfectly lovely kisser. Zero spark, but for my first date I think it was what I needed to ease into it all. We talked for quite a while after, even once I had said I wasn't sure there was a romantic future for us. Lovely, just lovely.

But, my friends, I wasn't there for lovely, was I? For the land of constant sex was dry. As dry as a bone and I wanted to get out there! And dating is, of course, the gateway to that. Being the full-throttle yet sensitive woman I am meant that I couldn't put myself in a sex-only situation at this point. Too vulnerable for that.

I went on a handful of dates in Manchester. I mean, I say "a handful," which is about right if you imagine the giant from *Jack and the Beanstalk* and think about the size of his hands. I was never friggin' at home!

One of my more formative experiences was with a boy I met who was from London and, of course, I found this exotic because I love a southern accent and I was still living up north at this point. The chat was literally the highlight of my days; we would talk nonstop, I found him hilarious, no dirty chat. The match happened because he was working up north a few times a week, staying in hotels. And so, after a couple of dates, I too would reside at said hotels with him. I was working as a physiotherapist at this time with the most amazing, supportive team that had handheld me through my breakup and they were so excited for me and my dating escapades. I would often go straight to work from the hotel, a two-hour commute. But, you know, anything for sex, connection, etc.

This one ended because he told me that he thought I wanted to be loved and that he didn't have the capacity to provide that for me. Fair enough. This was the first time I had felt the real void of my past relationship, I really missed feeling loved. Let's say this was a learning curve, but one that I would take absolutely no notice of. Onward.

Dicksand: quicksand, but for the love of penis

Then I found a lad who I saw for a good couple of months casually but we seemed to care for each other too, so it was the best of both worlds for a time. Then I got attached again. This attachment has been referred to as "dicksand" and I couldn't put it in a better way. Quicksand but with a penis.

I bought him a Christmas present and he shat his pants about it. We put some distance between us because, fair play to him, he was honest about not wanting anything more and could sense that I did. So we watched the DVD I bought him with not a single leg brush exchanged (I put a lot of pressure on these romantic, fleeting, hand-holding, leg-brushing moments)—it was *Frozen*, in case you were wondering. I now know that it is a rare thing to have a man be honest with you about his feelings and so, although it knocked my confidence a little, it was the most helpful thing for me. Dating isn't just about us and our feelings, there's another person in it with an entirely different history to us that will support and hinder the moves we make in different ways. Did I carry this learning with me into my next relationship though? No. I did not.

"There's no shame, only power, in the admission of knowing what you need and taking it."

He moved to London for work. We stayed in touch. Then I moved to London for work and he was a great friend to me when I arrived. By this point, I had moved on from the idea of him and I started my London dating career with some throttle. And guess what, lo and behold, he then wanted something more from ME! Pal, I'm in a new pool of men and I cannot be stopped, so let's just be friends?

London

London was an entirely different ball game, an infinite pool of men. I was new to the city and I was absolutely ready to throw myself into it all. There wasn't a single day in the week that I wasn't out on a date after work. Madness, but I absolutely thrived off it. I never got bored. It fixed my confidence up a treat and I think it's a powerful thing to admit that I needed men to help me with my wavering confidence at that time.

My dating career was something that defined me for a while. I was validated by the opposite sex. I needed that, though—the validation, the connection, to be desired by someone. These are all extremely normal feelings, especially when dating. It's a new landscape, new people and we aren't all built in the same way. That goes for all of you, too— there's no shame, only power, in the admission of knowing what you need and taking it. We're told time and time again that "you don't need a man to feel validated" and, hell, it's just not true for so many of us. My confidence in myself, my worth, and what I knew I wanted came back once I started to feel sexy and wanted again. (You're not allowed to beat yourself up if you aren't at that point yet; it'll come.)

The first pivotal dating relationship I experienced in London was with a man so handsome he hurt my eyes. Blonde, tall. Good grief. We met on a dating app and the chat was sporadic; I wasn't that fussed at first. We would reply whenever, with no pressure and no time constraints and the chat was great. Then, by way of an absolute curveball, he FACETIMED ME, drunk, from New York during a business trip and I have never applied makeup so quickly in my entire years of living. I was bang in trouble here; he was even more gorgeous than his photos. From this point, I could imagine what our kids might look like. Ahh fuck.

> *"The more experience that I have had, I now know what is driven by my vagina and what is driven by my heart."*

He was due to land back in London the next morning and he invited me round to his apartment. This was the date. At his apartment. I hadn't ever done this before and "stranger danger" is there to teach us not to turn up at boys' apartments for dates and sex if we don't know them. That said, I told my buddies the plan and it was the easiest yes

I'd given in a long time. If only you could have been inside my head to take note of the pure joy, excitement, anticipation, underwear options, and double shaving of legs to be nothing short of dolphin-like. This is a sneaky "dating" story really because, although we met on a dating app, we never, ever went on a date. You can imagine the setup. I used to even treat his injuries with physiotherapy from time to time. He was a triathlete (don't, you can't make it up). I'm going to leave this story here and I'll see you in the sex chapter for more on triathlete boy.

Sexual chemistry

There was another boy I got attached to. (I know this must be a shock.) He called me "Khaleesi" because at that time he was working on filming *Game of Thrones* and my hair was platinum blonde. You can imagine how much I loved the fact he had given me a nickname. This was another app match that resulted in our first date around at my apartment ... we both agreed not to murder each other and to order food and watch a movie. He stayed the night and we both passed comment on how well we got on, neither of us expecting any kind of connection beyond the sexual chemistry we had started with.

"I used to struggle with knowing what was love and what was lust."

We started to go out rather than just stay in and our dates were always so much fun. I thought he was really interesting, cool, intelligent, well dressed. But what a let down! He was one of those men who would make a plan then break it an hour before. He did this to me on my birthday, exactly an hour before I was due to see him and I hadn't ever felt quite so sad as I did climbing back into bed with full hair and makeup done and proceeding to order myself a pizza. The thing is, he didn't owe me anything; he wasn't my boyfriend and the sadness I felt came from the pressure I had put on seeing someone I was casually dating on my birthday. He was one of those ones that you keep in your phone book for times of sex-drought safe in the knowledge that good sex is all you will get and nothing more.

Holiday weekend

This next dating story is an absolute joke. It started out with the best chat, jokes, and wit ever over the app. In actual fact, a friend of mine matched with him for me, started the chat, and I had to pick up where her smart remarks left off. It was a holiday weekend and there were some day festivals happening; I was at one, he was at another. We agreed to meet up afterward in a local bar. The spark was great, the right amount of flirty, fun. I bought the drinks. We got more and more drunk and I had plans to be at a friend's afterward and, brave as he was, he came with me.

He fit right in, didn't need babysitting. Then he came up to me and asked me to lend him $55 cash until he went to an ATM and so, deep in conversation, I gave it to him, not really paying attention to what it might be for. I didn't know until about a week later that it was for drugs. I found out when I got a phone call from what I can only describe as a dealer who was owed $55 … This guy hadn't used the $55 I gave him to pay said dealer for his drugs and so I paid the dealer. Mortified. I mean, this is ridiculous—even typing it out, I'm laughing. There were people I didn't know at this party who, it seemed, liked to "dabble" in substances beyond alcohol.

Somehow he made it seem like nothing, saying he would pay me back and he was so sorry, making light of it all. He was so much fun that I kind of just brushed it off. We talked a lot, saw each other on and off when we had time. The turning point came when we were at my friend's wedding and he let the mother of the bride (who he did not know) BUY HIM A DRINK. WHY DID HE NOT BUY HER A DRINK? The mother of the bride is the most amazing woman who I have known my entire life. I was livid about it. After the wedding, we went our separate ways, I got drunk at a Bastille gig, sent him a voicemail containing lyrics about not being good enough, and closed the book on him. What a ride. Never got my fucking $55 back either. Or the $55 I paid to the dealer. So there I am $110 short, and still no prospective husband.

♦

I want to end my part of the dating chapter by talking about love. Taking the leap from dating someone when it's gone in the best possible way, leading you to fall absolutely head over heels in L.O.V.E. The feeling of falling in love. Oh, what a joy this is. My favorite thing in the world is to be in love.

What I like most about the journey into goo-goo-eyed town is the mixed bag of feelings and finally a crescendo that presents itself before you. I used to struggle with knowing what was love and what was lust—because for me, both feelings made my head fall off and forget my own name. The older I've become and more experience that I have had, I now know exactly what is driven by my vagina and what is driven by my heart.

I always think that you know you're in love when you feel things for a person that you don't feel for anyone else. You're willing to take the rough with the smooth—their wonderful qualities and the ones that make you want to commit a small murder. Either way, they are the person you don't want to go through life without, the person you miss the most when you're apart.

The moment you realize you're in love with someone is really quite special; it might have hit you as they are lacing up their shoes up in a way that makes no logical sense, it might be the way they supported you through something. It can be overwhelming, especially if it's an unspoken love at this point; you can't just go blurting it out but you also can't keep it to yourself. We often build it up into quite the declaration, which works for me. I love a big show of emotion! But not all of us do, so just take it easy and show it in a way that suits you.

Now that you've fallen in love, congratulations, welcome to the aforementioned goo-goo-eyed town. But being in love is a different kettle of fish, filled with ups and downs, some heavy questions, and memories that you'll cherish forever and ever Amen. Love, as they say, is often about compromise and is absolutely not a straight road. To maintain happiness in love, you've got to be able to ride it all together, be there, be supportive, trust each other. I don't know a single couple who are in love and do not argue. It's a myth, just in case you had heard otherwise! Life is tricky, as we know—this entire book is based on the fact and things aren't going to be rosy 100 percent of the time. It's what you do with the hard parts that makes you stronger. Love will grow in different ways over time, too. We move forward from the honeymoon period and into a deeper, more developed level of love as you begin to learn more and more about the other person. I don't think learning about one another in this way will ever reach an end as we all evolve so much over the course of our lives.

I have fallen in what I thought was love quite a few times— as, like I said, I used to struggle to separate lust and love. One of my favorite love stories is this: an online match that would last and last. Two people who were trying to do things differently, take each other seriously, not rush into things, or into bed (we failed on that last one). Those first months where nothing stands in the way of you making plans to spend time together are just the best; you get to know each other intimately and gobble up one another's life story. That's when the love came, when I truly started to understand this person and liked them more as I learned.

Then one day, lying in bed watching a Scandinavian drama, preparing for our first week apart since we met three months ago, we both roll over to face each other and there's a loaded silence that fills the air, and his eyes. The "I love yous" come tumbling out and I think my heart might stop. This is my favorite love story.

Lizzy on **Dating**

I am not a natural dater. I can't flirt for the life of me and my reaction to someone flirting with me is just as awkward to witness. It literally causes a bright red rash to slowly grow from my neck onto my cheeks. Needless to say, it's very sexy. I watch other people flirt (Lindsey, this is directed at you) and just cannot get my head around the subtlety of it, how someone moves from speaking normally to suddenly advancing to something flirtatious. It's a skill I do not possess.

This also transfers into the digital world, it turns out. I once had a boyfriend who admitted that my dry humor sometimes didn't come across so well over a message until you really got to know me, which makes me think I could send men bolting for the door at the first sarcastic message. It makes the whole process of dating rather stressful at times. Ultimately, I have decided to just embrace all of this and hope to the high heavens that the flirt-rash could possibly be seen as sort of cute and endearing? We live in hope for that one anyway.

I think the whole concept of dating apps is amazing; I love the fact you can sit on your couch at home and meet people you would otherwise have never crossed paths with. And the truth of living in London is that people don't really talk to one another too often and it's hard to actually meet people "in real life." But I still think you have to be in a healthy headspace for it to be a healthy experience. Sometimes that definitely can be when you're trying to get over someone but you have to be realistic about where you are at and what you want from someone. Want to date to sleep around and enjoy exploring yourself and your sexuality? Go. For. It. Want to date to sleep around to make someone jealous? Maybe not so wise. Want to date to meet new people and make new connections? I can't think of anything better than the apps. Desperately searching for validation through a new relationship without actually owning or understanding that? It will likely put too much pressure on someone else. The whole thing is a learning curve and takes some mistakes to eventually get it right; by which I mean, to get to a point where the experiences (even the bad ones) are healthy and fun and not causing any long-term sadness aside from the standard "he didn't text me back" woes.

The age-old "you'll meet someone when you least expect it" definitely has some truth in it! When I started dating my ex, who I met in real life a few years prior to us ever actually taking a step further with anything, I wasn't looking for anything new. It turned out to be the best sort of dating possible. We made it a rather global affair, due to him living in another country, and it was everything dating should feel like. Lots of fun, initially not too much pressure at all, getting to know one another at a pace that suited us both, and introducing one another to new things and people as we went. Long distance actually has a lot of perks too—it means you get your own time (very important for me) when you're both in your own cities and you always have something look forward to, whenever you are going to see each other next. As he is an ex, of course it didn't work out in the long run, but the experience of the beginning few months was incredible fun and something I look back on with so much fondness.

When you meet someone new it can really open your life up to so much—all the people, interests, and experiences another person holds that then become available to you. Isn't that so amazing? I think there is so much to be said for this stage in a relationship outside of all of the passion and butterflies—just the meeting and sharing of two lives is so exciting, no matter how long it lasts. It's something that I would definitely hope to experience again in my life and this really changed my outlook on dating after the aforementioned not-so-great experiences!

"It's scary knowing you're walking into territory that might leave you hurting. But I do recommend you walk in."

Dating goes beyond the first few times you meet someone or swiping through the apps. It is the starting point of a relationship that can move in a whole host of directions. But sometimes the tricky bit can be getting something off the ground, deciding if you even want to, or the agony of mixed signals from another person. I do stand by the idea that a mixed signal is a clear signal in itself, as if someone wants you they will make it known, but at the same time, I do also appreciate it's not that black and white sometimes. There is a whole host of things to consider: your attachment style (learning about this was a game changer for me and something I will come back to), what is going on in the other person's life at the time, your own standards of communication, your own love language. And all of these can come to the surface within just days or weeks of meeting someone.

The immediacy of communication nowadays is a blessing and a curse. It can make a slow reply time feel excruciating and there are so many ways to find out if and when the person was online and torture yourself with that information. Not everything is love at first sight (actually, in my experience, it never is), so there is a messy bit of groundwork that goes into the beginning stages that can take up huge amounts of energy—but also be very exciting!

One of my own experiences with getting past the initial dating stage is a perfect example of why timing is everything. It was with my ex, who had done his fair share of dating in his time! We had met years before the first night we got together, which came about totally spontaneously after he invited me out with his friends. Due to him living abroad, there was little guarantee of when we would see each other again. I wasn't really ready for a relationship as I was still dealing with lots of things from past relationships. This meant I ended up playing it really aloof for the first few months.

"You have to be prepared to do the work here and learn how to communicate."

I use the word "playing" reluctantly here because I wasn't playing a game and I am the sort of person who cannot pretend not to be interested—I go all in. At this time, it wasn't for a lack of interest in this person, more down to a lack of capacity to build on something just then. This, predictably, made him a hundred times more interested in me! While I don't think game playing is a good idea (unless you are strong enough to really play the long game), this was a real lightbulb moment of realizing how much people do want what feels slightly out of reach. It all came to a head with a very frank conversation led by him outlining what he wanted and openly asking me what was going on with me. And we went on to have a very happy and fun relationship for almost a year.

This story I think demonstrates perfectly how much goes on with people when you first meet; there can be so much that makes things incredibly complicated. But the key thing in that experience was communication. It does have to be in a timely fashion—if you are saying "WHAT ARE WE?!" after one date, that may well go down like a lead balloon. But there comes a certain point when you're dating that you have to be brave and have the conversation. If you are agonizing over it every day as you fall deeper in love, you aren't likely to be feeling overwhelmingly happy. And I know how scary the thought of hearing what you don't want to hear can be but, in the long run, it will prove the right thing to have done because you will be able to make decisions based on knowledge and not your own musings, which I think in these situations can be wildly incorrect.

The balance of going into something with an open mind and heart while also protecting the most vulnerable parts of yourself is perhaps the biggest crux of falling in love. You cannot control other people and yet in those moments when your feelings are intensifying, it's all you want to be able to do. It's scary knowing you're walking into territory that might leave you hurting. But I do always recommend you walk in. I have made the mistake many times of walking in a little TOO eagerly and bringing every part of myself with me and very visibly on show. It has ended in huge amounts of pain, but ultimately I wouldn't change it, as I have learned a lot from it.

I will come back to the lessons I have learned soon, but what about the dream scenario where you meet someone and it's effortless? You are both on the same page, timing has worked entirely in your favor, the two of you are ready to jump in with both feet. Especially when you meet someone where you just have that spark, you have so much fun, there is so much to talk about, the sex is amazing and, slowly and surely, all those feelings of love start to develop. It has to be one of the best parts of life, when those feelings first start to grow and become more intense. When it seems an effort to keep the rest of your life ticking along because really you just want to drop off the map and solely be with your person (it's very important that you don't!). The honeymoon period of a relationship is just pure bliss. But getting past that is what can be tricky. It's where my last relationship fell down, and where many do.

I thrive in something that brings me security, so I actually love the transition. But for others it can be scary and the natural doubts that come up about a person who, up until that moment, has (unsustainably) felt like the best thing since sliced bread, get louder and louder until they tell you to leave. You have to be prepared to do the work here and learn how to communicate things that will help you navigate the inevitable change of pace the relationship is about to experience. Two people coming together and deciding to build their life together is hard work, when you think of all the aspects that have to align, all the compromises that come up along the way. But hard work doesn't mean an unhappy life; hard work can be so, so fulfilling. And the important distinction is that all the hard work isn't just coming from you with no reward but from both parties, with the goal being to make each other happy.

The most useful thing I learned recently was about attachment styles from the brilliant book *Attached* by Amir Levine and Rachel S. F. Heller. I think understanding your own attachment style is essential when meeting someone new but also when you're in an established relationship. According to Levine and Heller, the three recognized styles of attachment are: anxious, avoidant, and secure. A general overview is that you secure lot have got it good and can generally respond well to either an anxious or avoidant partner: if they withdraw slightly, you don't panic; if they need reassurance over something, you are comfortable giving it. The most difficult, of course, is the anxious–avoidant combination. The avoidant withdraws in some way as they feel pressure to emotionally commit; the anxious person is highly sensitive to this and so pursues them for the reassurance; the avoidant sees that as more pressure and retreats further and the anxious person becomes more anxious. As someone with an anxious attachment, this made *so* much sense to me and gave me so much clarity in what I should look for in a partner and why previous "anxious–avoidant traps" I found myself in were incredibly hard to break. You are both responding in a way that's instinctive to you, and to overcome that is obviously a challenge. It isn't all doom and gloom, of course, but I think the best takeaway for me was the understanding of why something feels so triggering sometimes. This means that you can at least communicate with yourself much better, and in turn with others.

LOVE OR LUST?

As Lindsey said: are you thinking with your vagina or are you thinking with your heart? Love is a messy feeling that can be impossible to pull apart, especially when it comes to distinguishing between love and infatuation, so for help, start by asking yourself these questions:

A loving relationship gives you space to live your own life too and doing so shouldn't make you an anxious mess. Do you feel like all your energy is taken up by your other half, so you don't have much left over for yourself?

Yes □   No □

Sex is an important part of any relationship but does yours have lots of positive aspects beyond the bedroom too? Does most of the time you spend with each other revolve around sleeping together?

Yes □   No □

Aside from the time spent together that does revolve around sex, is the relationship based on sexual chemistry as opposed to shared values and interests? Basically, is the main thing you have in common that you like to sleep with each other?

Yes □   No □

Do you feel stuck in a cycle of extreme highs and lows? It can be easy to mistake this for an intense connection but it's often more likely to be a result of some toxicity within the relationship.

Yes ☐ No ☐

Do you have a habit of jumping ship as soon as a relationship ends the honeymoon period? Do you feel that familiar itch in this relationship?

Yes ☐ No ☐

If you answered "yes" to most of these, signs point toward it being an infatuation rather than a deep, loving connection. Or perhaps you are even mistaking the addiction to an up-and-down relationship for true chemistry. That isn't to say infatuation can't be a part of that connection but it has to be built on more than simply lust to be sustainable. A toxic relationship can be the hardest kind to remove yourself from, or even recognize at times, as its intensity is likely to be unmatched by any other relationship you have had before. But you must remind yourself that steadiness is actually such a blessing in life because it gives you the space to explore other parts of yourself and your interests with a loving relationship as a foundation. An infatuation will likely absorb a lot of your energy and may often leave you feeling confused about aspects of the relationship.

It's not all doom and gloom though. These experiences are so important for you to have under your belt to understand more of what you want from love!

LINDSEY'S TOP TIPS FOR DATING AND FLIRTING IN THE FLESH

(For Lizzy to read and take note of also)

Right, I'm no guru but I've also never been as dry as a bone once I started dating, so I've got to be doing something right—or at least, not terribly wrong. Neither dating nor flirting used to come naturally to me, so it's been a body of work (my body) that has taken years of practice, years of Dutch courage.

In short, you've got to be ready to just say "fuck it" and go and get the person you want. Let them know you want them. Dating is a tricky business because statistics suggest you will meet a lot of weirdos before you meet someone you can get drunk and have a relatively good conversation with. Trust me, the flash on my camera has outed me while trying to take a sneaky photo of my date to caption "HE IS NOTHING LIKE HIS PHOTO" and send to my friends.

> *"We are romantics at heart who can throw all caution to the wind for love, or sometimes even just a night of passion."*

My general rule of thumb for dating, specifically online dating, is to build up some fun and thriving conversations over a period of a week or two so you know at least 4 percent of the person before walking in to find out they are in fact part horse. You will know as soon as you clap eyes on them whether there is a sexual—or any!—attraction there. I always find that if it's not there at the start it won't build for me.

Dating after meeting in real life often comes off the back of a flirt. So let's talk about how to flirt. God, this is hysterical, like something out of the 1950s: "Flirting to Catch Your Man." Step 1: Wear your best petticoat.

So seriously, for me it's all in the eyes. Eye contact is the quickest, most efficient way to let the other person know you're interested in them. Holding eye contact for a couple of seconds is quite a long time. Try it now: look at something for two seconds. Then look away fairly slowly to show you're not sorry you've been caught staring. With any luck, this is taken as an invitation for them to come and chat to you; if not, head over there and start the conversation yourself.

You can start with anything, my Dutch courage helps me out in this department. I'd usually say something like "good shirt"—a compliment, but not too much. (I am aware that this is like the start of a bad rom com. The irony isn't lost on me.) It just needs to be something short to open up a conversation, exchange of drinks and numbers, and away you go! You can either set the pace for the chat or decide to let them lead, whatever makes you feel more comfortable. Flirting isn't lap dances and "come to bed eyes"—although it *is* in the eyes. It's confidence in yourself and a wry smile.

DATING TIPS FROM A PERSON WHO GETS A RASH ON THEIR NECK WHEN SOMEONE FLIRTS WITH THEM (LIZZY)

Just reading Lindsey's tips makes me feel the rash starting to come up. I honestly felt blotchy trying to hold eye contact with a pen pot as practice, so I am sure if it was another person I would look like I was midway through some dramatic allergic reaction.

I have seen Linds in action before and wanted to share a great example of such a moment. We were at a press event, and they often hire catering staff that look like models (probably are models) at this sort of thing. Lindsey had already had the eye-contact moment with one of them and so he, of course, kept coming over with his tray of canapés—meaning the rest of us were benefiting in the form of tiny burgers. Then the guy came out with tray of (mini) desserts and explained to us what they were. I can't remember what it was but I do remember us all saying we didn't like it. Now, I know Linds' dietary requirements like the back of my hand and this was definitely *not* up her alley. Despite that, she said: "Oh gosh, maybe, do you like it? Do you recommend it?"—all eye contact with this guy. We all fell about laughing and said, "Hang on a minute, was our opinion not enough here?!" Lindsey continued her chat with this fella over a dessert I know full well she hated. It was all just innocent flirting that went no further and she was totally unfazed even by the rest of us all laughing so hard over the whole thing. My rash could have had me hospitalized at that stage if it had been me.

How far will we go for love?

As you may have guessed, we are both romantics at heart who can throw all caution to the wind for love, or sometimes even just a night of passion. We will leave it to you to guess who did what here—answers are at the very end of the book (on page 216).

1 Who used to do a four-hour commute to work just to be able to see their boyfriend overnight?

Lindsey □   Lizzy □

2 Who once paid almost $138 for an emergency dermatologist appointment to get rid of an ingrown hair that cropped up just weeks before seeing a boy she had fancied for ages?

Lindsey □   Lizzy □

3 Who once spent hours burning a CD for a boy she fancied and then drawing all over it, scratching it to bits so that it wouldn't even play?

Lindsey □   Lizzy □

4   Who cut off all her long hair into a near-on pixie crop
    for a boy?

    Lindsey ☐   Lizzy ☐

5   Who used to go home after a night out, go to sleep for
    a few hours, then drive to pick up a boy from the same
    club when he rang to bring him back to her uni halls?

    Lindsey ☐   Lizzy ☐

6   Who pretended to be really chilled about hearing
    about a boy's previous girlfriends/dates at the
    beginning of a relationship when really they felt like
    their insides were on fire?

    Lindsey ☐   Lizzy ☐

7   Who took out two separate overdrafts to be able to
    afford to go to Australia to see her boyfriend?

    Lindsey ☐   Lizzy ☐

8   Who once pretended she wanted to learn how to play
    the bass guitar so she could have "lessons" from a boy
    in high school?

    Lindsey ☐   Lizzy ☐

9 Who turned up to her boyfriend's workplace—a local grocery store—and proposed to him with a letter after she kissed someone else on a girls' vacation?

Lindsey ☐   Lizzy ☐

10 Who collected crystals to give out to boys she liked in school as "love beads"? The first lucky recipient was called Martin.

Lindsey ☐   Lizzy ☐

CHAPTER 6

Sex

Welcome to the fun chapter! Have you ever taken a photo of a man sleeping next to you to send to your best friend? Have you ever had sex in a hotel lobby bathroom because you couldn't wait to get to the room? Either yes or no in answer to those questions is totally fine, but we are here to tell you that we have and we are not shy about saying we both love sex. It's such a fun part of life and so many good memories and even better stories can come out of these escapades (sexcapades, if you will). Whatever stage you're at in your own sexual journey, it can be so reassuring and sometimes just downright fun to listen to other people's experiences. In a part of our lives that is so intimate, it's lovely to know there are so many similarities we all experience.

Lindsey on Sex

Mom and Dad, please, I beg you, skip this chapter!
(The same applies to anyone who has known me since
I was little.)

I wasn't always a promiscuous woman. It hit me at
college off the back of some male attention that I'd never
experienced before. This unlocked my sexuality, passion,
and erm, increasingly high sex drive.

Sex can be incredibly empowering but also render you a bit
powerless where emotion is concerned, when you start to
fall for a person.

As women, the narrative around us and sex can be
somewhat negative. If you like sex or have a lot of sex with
multiple partners, say, you could have found yourself labeled
"the local slut" or "easy." This, my friends, is simply not
the case, so if you've ever been made to feel this way, and
I know I have, it's absolutely untrue and you are a goddess.
Sex is a wonderful thing and, as long as we are choosing
to use our bodies in that way with no pressure attached,
in circumstances that are always completely consensual,
it's one of the most powerful things to create intimacy, no
matter the level of relationship you may or may not be in.
Sex and your sexuality is about finding out what you like
and the exploration of your own body, which is yours to use
however you damn well like. Regardless of how many sexual
partners you have.

I've had some bad sex in my time, we all have. Usually owing to a drunken night of passion that creeps up on you, regardless of the quick shave you did prenight out just in case.

One scenario that really sticks with me is the time I took a boy home at uni. We had fancied each other for a while after seeing each other on various student nights out and I had given him all my best sultry eye contact, never speaking to each other, until now.

It was one of those kissing up the side of a wall on the way home, not really drawing breath type connections. All sexual. We fell through the door of my university dorms, collapsed onto the bed, I kissed him some more and (I swear that this is one of my greatest achievements ever) he came in his boxers. Well, well, well. That was the end of that. At 19 years old I wasn't equipped to deal with such a finish, so I reassured him it was fine, went to the bathroom, had a quick laugh, and went back to bed.

I didn't see him again.

Sex on a girls' vacation can be a rite of passage for so many of us and, again, it's never anything to be ashamed of. We're all out here exploring, having fun, and as long as we're safe there's really nothing to discuss. Enjoy every experience, learn about your body, know your limits and the power of control too. The way you use your body is always up to you; if it's safe and feels good then go for it.

Girls' vacation sex is always up there with some of the worst: you're the most drunk, your radar is ever so slightly off due to a constant state of intoxication owing to the cheap booze on offer, and then there's the hot climate and thrush to contend with. I met a boy I liked, and even liked him sober. I met him around the pool of our apartments. All the boys in his group and all the girls in my group got together; it was the best fun. Everyone pairing off, kissing and being fingered on the dance floor (not me on this occasion).

> *"Here she is again, the woman who is unable to separate sex from emotion. Will she ever learn? The answer is no, absolutely not."*

We spent a night together and a few things happened. There was a burning fire between my legs and not because I was enthralled by him, it was thrush. I came on my period (WHY NOW? YOU WEREN'T DUE TO BE HERE!) and my hands turned red and swelled up to around three times their usual size. I said this during a podcast episode and I'll say it again: hell hath no fury like a woman with thrush. I can't even tell you what the sex was like because I was so wrapped up in all the ailments that were appearing before my eyes. I snuck out of his bed and went to my own in the middle of the night and we didn't speak about the sex again. Nor have any more.

During your sexual career, you will meet people who have certain quirks, fantasies, things you may not be used to in bed. This story is a mild version of just that.

Fast forward to my first few months in London and I had matched with a handsome guy on a dating app. We went for drinks, got on well, he was an even bigger flirt than I am and he was blowing my mind. For our second date, I found myself in an Uber to his house at 11 p.m. On a school night. I often did this, threw caution to the wind and decided to enjoy every drop of whatever I wanted to. Let it be known I was also very tired during this spell in my life!

We're watching a movie in bed, messing around a bit and then he whispered something. I couldn't quite hear him so I asked again. "Lick my nipples." Sorry, what? "Lick my nipples, please." Oh for fuck's sake. I laughed and did it anyway, and never saw him again. That may have been your thing, pal, but it was not mine. Didn't even know his surname. Sir Licks-a-nipple.

I don't think I have any quirks except maybe things like not wearing any panties on my way to see the man I'm off to have the ride of my life with. And maybe that this man asked me not to wear the panties and to keep them in my back pocket.

Which leads me nicely into my next fun escapade. Remember triathlete boy from my dating chapter? Him. It was him.

So the sex with him was like nothing I had ever experienced in my life up until that point. There were absolutely no boundaries, which in turn meant there wasn't a shred of embarrassment between us. Two passionate people letting each other know exactly what the deal was.

Now, I've already told you that him and I never, ever went on any dates. It was all at his apartment, it was all sex, and movies, and wine. Oh and some physio treatment ahead of his races. The passion remained in my head, near on drowning me when I was apart from him. From sending NSFW (not safe for work) photos to him during our working days, to not being able to think about anything else except that good, good love and the next time I would get it.

"Always trust your body and go with the flow."

On one particular occasion, I was out for some drinks with the girls and I got a text from him asking what I was doing and if I was free would I like to come over? But a little more explicit than that. You get the idea. My stomach flipped. I gave it ten minutes then responded to say I was out for drinks but would see if I could come by after. Knowing full well I was going to reapply my lipstick and leave immediately. His next text message was a request: "Take off your panties, put them in your back pocket now." So, of course I whipped them off. I was wearing a skirt and had to get the metro, FYI. I have never clamped my legs together so hard. What we didn't want was a reenactment of *Basic Instinct* on the train line.

I arrived, the door barely shut behind me and I was up against a cupboard in the entrance to his apartment. Gosh, I feel like I'm writing an erotic novel.

All of our encounters were like this, full of passion. I never wanted it to stop. I wanted to spend my life on the other end of sex, from him. (I was going to write, "spend my life on the other end of his penis" but then I thought that might be too much?)

I think this all-consuming feeling also came from a place I didn't want it to: I really, really liked him. Here she is again, the woman who is unable to separate sex from emotion. Will she ever learn? The answer is no, absolutely not.

Lindsey's letter to her virgin self

Listen. I'm just going to get right to it. Your first time will be on the bathroom floor of a stranger's house party and you will both be too nervous and too wasted to do anything with that blueberry condom. Spit it out. You don't know how to give a blow job yet.

Your virginity is precious, yes, but don't put so much pressure on yourself. You've got a beautiful body, even though you don't really know how to shave your pubes. Or what shape they're supposed to take on?

After many months of obsessing over sex and being fingered in the build up to it, it will disappoint you, it will not set off fireworks in your panties. You will bleed, it will hurt, you will panic that you got pregnant on the first go.

However, it does get better. Much better, in fact, but it will not get better until you start to experiment with your body and with someone you trust. You will buy all manner of things from various shopping mall sexual pleasure stores, not limited to tingling balms—though do yourself a favor and leave those well alone after the first incident. There is such a thing as too much tingle.

You will have a lot of sex when in search of your sexuality and what works for you. Your friends will be very proud of your "number" for you. You will have sex around the world, which is very exciting and, erm, enlightening. This does not mean you are a slutty-slut girl. Just try not to have sex with multiple people from the same friendship group as a starting point ...

If there was one piece of advice I could share with you it would be to always trust your body and to go with the flow— to find out so much about your body is a truly special thing so enjoy every moment, even the experiences that are over way too quickly!

LIZZY ON Sex

I once had a one-night stand after which I have never left a hotel room so fast in my life. It all started in Paris. Linds and I were having dinner and a very handsome older man sitting next to us started up a conversation. We all ended up heading to a bar for some drinks, sharing life stories in that way you do when you're a few cocktails in, and feel like you need to get to know a stranger in record-breaking time.

On about the fourth Old Fashioned, I decided my intentions were clear in my mind: I was going back to this man's hotel room. After quickly asking Lindsey to touch my leg and let me know if it felt too hairy, we decided that this was a grown man and if he was going to run off at the sight of a slightly hairy leg and vagina then he wouldn't be missed. Lindsey made her goodbyes and headed back to our hotel room, I made it clear to her I wasn't planning on sleeping over (make of that what you will, I hate the thought of waking up next to someone unless I do have some sort of feelings for them aside from "you're fit").

"There is huge joy in the discovery of someone's body and preferences."

As a side note here—a friend once told me a brilliant line for either making your goodbyes if you've gone back to theirs or getting them out of your place: "I've got a barbecue in Cambridge at ten." The perfect amount of detail, the perfect distance from London, and one that can be used year-round, because even in the depths of winter, it sounds too specific to be a lie. (Though I couldn't possibly make it back to Cambridge for 10 a.m. from Paris, so this excuse was made redundant for that night.)

Anyway, off we go back to his hotel and proceed to have some of the least satisfactory sex of my life! He was quite a bit older than me so I was thinking I was in for the experienced older man. But alas, I did not hit that jackpot. I didn't even make any excuses. We sat and discussed Freudian theory for a bit (the most stimulating part of the night) and then I just announced I was leaving and left so quickly that I didn't even have my shoelaces done up when I walked back into mine and Lindsey's hotel room.

So, judging by that story, you can assume I am not shy of casual sex from time to time. Even though it wasn't particularly satisfying, the entire night was so much fun and the whole experience of meeting someone new is always enjoyable. When you are in a headspace that can take sex as *just sex*, something fun for both parties, then I think there is no place for judgment at all for a one-night stand! So long as your mental health isn't being negatively affected, then get your fill whenever and with whomever you fancy.

Casual hookups can be so much fun and provide great stories to retell at parties but my experiences have always reinforced that the best sex you will have is when there is an emotional connection there. I think this is where we can often fall down with our intentions of keeping something casual—unless the feelings *don't* develop, the more you get to know someone, the better the sex seems to get. It's like all the layers of intimacy come together to just make the physical connection all the more special. I have found I am one extreme to the next—either "barbecue in Cambridge at ten and please don't ever contact me again" or "I will die for you and spend months and months trying to get over you, and then I still might not manage it." And it's as soon as I really invest in someone that I am in hook, line, and sinker. It's an intoxicating mix of so many emotions and the reason I have never had a one-night stand that matches up with the feeling of getting into bed with someone who you are connected to on levels beyond the physical attraction. There is such a huge amount of joy in the discovery of someone's body and preferences, alongside getting to know their personality.

"It's important to understand how fragile a libido can be. If you're having a day, a week, a month, without a sex drive it's not time to become a nun."

This, of course, mostly applies to the first year of being with someone, the overwhelming butterflies as you discover more and more of a person. When you are in a long-term relationship, there is, of course, a moment when this plateaus, when you feel like you have discovered all you could know about someone and things in the bedroom can slip into routine, or even into nonexistence.

> "It's unrealistic to think that things will always be fireworks and rose-tinted glasses."

This is where the discovery of one another has to become more purposeful and can't rely on all the endorphins that are released in the first few months of a relationship. It's a moment when lots of relationships might fail, as we can run from one to the next constantly searching for that passion again. But, of course, it can be found without jumping ship from your relationship; it just takes a realistic appraisal of what actually happens as you become more and more familiar with someone. And it doesn't have to feel like the beginning of the end, rather the beginning of a new phase of a relationship, that almost every couple will experience.

What was once exciting is now predictable; when they were once perfect they are now highly irritating; what was once sexy is now try-hard. As we discussed in the breakups chapter, there are, of course, moments when you will have to decide if these feelings are accompanied by others that do signify it's time to say goodbye. But it's also unrealistic to think that things will always be fireworks and rose-tinted glasses. It's also important to understand how fragile a libido can be at times. If you're having a day, a week, a month, without a sex drive it's not time to run to the hills and become a nun. Equally, if your partner is going through that, try not to take it incredibly personally.

There is so much that affects your libido: stress, tiredness, low self-esteem, depression, or even less extreme bouts of poor mental health, and that's just to name a few.

> *"You will learn what a fun, joyful and happy thing sex can be in your life."*

A sex drive can ebb and flow and it's important to try to focus a lot on your own mood and happiness around it rather than imagining what everyone else might be up to. Haven't had sex for a few weeks but you're both very happy and know you're just missing your mojo? Then ride it out, until you're *literally* riding it out again. Noticing you're in a dry spell for longer because the thought of having sex with your partner is becoming unbearable (maybe you feel like their mom or are loving them too much like a best friend, as really it has now just become a friendship)? Then it's time to address the bigger picture.

Sex in our lives is a journey of highs and lows. From dreadful one-night stands to the wild throes of a new relationship, to the routine of knowing just *how* to give someone pleasure when you've been with them for years. But there really is joy in all of those moments.

Lizzy's letter to her virgin self

You, like every other teenager, feel in a rush to experience certain things. And while it's very easy for me to look back and tell you that you don't need to feel rushed, those feelings were there at the time for a reason. You were in a hurry to feel grown-up, to experience things other people were and to avoid feeling like you were being left behind. With hindsight, you will see how unimportant all of these things actually are but in the moment it really did matter! Thankfully, that sense of urgency didn't lead you to make any choices you have lived to regret.

Most of your first sexual experiences coincided with when your dad is quite poorly and you incidentally have quite considerable memory loss over a two-year period between the ages of 16 and 18. Losing your virginity will feel like a huge deal at the time but you're not going to be able to recall it one bit (honestly, you can barely remember a single thing about it)! But that's not something that bothers you; it's just one of those things and was due to your life at the time. Plus you have lots more fun sex coming up, so don't fret about that.

You will go through a phase when you are in a relationship for many years that you feel judgment of other people sleeping around. This isn't good and you won't look back on that proudly (not that you ever voiced it, thank goodness!). In hindsight, it was probably a subconscious jealousy of what others were experiencing at the time.

The niggle of wanting to experience more sexual partners will grow in your relationship as your desire for that person dwindles. It's a painful time and you spend a lot of it denying your own sexual desires in an attempt to convince yourself to stay in the relationship, but eventually you make the right decision. You will feel sad about it for many years, but there is a learning experience there too because you realize that sadness doesn't necessarily mean you did something wrong. The grass was greener and you have some great stories to tell from making such a brave jump. It is one of the times when you really successfully listened to your body, head, and heart!

From that point on, there will be one-night stands. There will be some incredible connections and you will meet people who you are more comfortable with than you could ever imagine. You will learn what a fun, joyful, and happy thing sex can be in your life.

Don't worry too much about it, or overthink it, you have so many amazing experiences ahead!

QUESTIONS AND ANSWERS: SEX

As this chapter has hopefully demonstrated, anyone's sex life is full of lots of ups and downs (no pun intended). We remember when we first started talking about sex a lot with friends. It was normally at predrinks before a night out, while covering ourselves with fake tan that was about to streak in the rain, false eyelashes hanging off in one corner and jabbing you in the eye, the overpowering smell of hairspray in the room, and a horrifyingly strong vodka and coke in hand. At the time, lots of us were having our first sexual experiences, so, of course, it would be the hottest topic of conversation: "How much do you shave?! What's the right amount?", "Oh wow, it does taste like that, doesn't it?!", "I got some raspberry-flavored lube from Ann Summers too!"

In adult life, it may not often come up in conversation with quite the same vigor. As people fall into established relationships, it can feel more and more personal to discuss. It's not just funny stories of us all finding our way now but an intimate thing between two people that everyone has the right to keep private. But despite that, it's a big part of life, so it must always feel OK to discuss when you need to, which is where we come in …

I have never had sex. How do I choose the right person?

Lizzy: So long as you feel safe and respected, that's about as right as it's going to get. It's never going to be great and there are advantages to it being both of your first times (new territory for you both can make it feel less intimidating!) and to your partner having a little more experience (maybe to make you feel more relaxed). Discovering your sexual self is a journey that doesn't begin and end with losing your virginity, so try not to put too much pressure on yourself over it. The important parts are to look after your mental and sexual health—knowing you feel "ready" emotionally is the thing that only you can decide and the main bit to listen to yourself on.

Lindsey: Don't force anything in this department—as you've probably read earlier in the chapter, blueberry condoms and losing your virginity do not mix. It will happen for you and you'll know when you meet the right person too. Make sure it's on your terms and that you're safe. (Condoms yes, it's the blueberry flavor that's optional.) Explore on your own too and figure out what you like so you're not waiting for someone to provide the pleasure. That's also a fun part!

How do you navigate the differences in sex drives in a relationship?

Lizzy: This can definitely be such a hard thing to talk about but it is something that every couple will come up against at some point. The first thing to do is know it's normal not to always be on the same page with your libido. The second thing is to be really honest with yourself when a lack of sex drive becomes actually not having any sexual attraction to that person for a sustained period of time. So much affects our libido: stress, depression, tiredness, low self-esteem, emotional worry. It can be hard being on either end of this situation—the one pursuing sex and feeling rejected or the one denying sex and questioning themselves.

This is why you have to communicate and not let it turn into something that bubbles away and suddenly becomes a lot bigger. A simple, "I've noticed we haven't had sex as much recently and it's making me worried a little, is everything OK with you? Have you noticed this too?" Or, "I realized we aren't having sex as often and I think it's down to how I am feeling. I am just stressed/feeling low/not feeling like myself (whichever is applicable) and, as a result, my sex drive doesn't feel normal, but I promise this isn't anything to do with you and I will keep speaking openly about it."

However, it's really important not to start this conversation if this has just been a one-night thing—your partner doesn't always have to be in the mood just because you are—but if you notice it going on for a while (and however long that is depends on what is "normal" for you both in your relationship) then don't let it sit under the surface.

The other scenario is when you know you're just not feeling it with that person anymore. It can be so easy to put this down to all the reasons we know genuinely do affect your sex drive, especially when you've been together for a long time. But if you really just don't want to have sex with that person anymore and are giving false excuses when they ask about it, it's time to be honest with them and yourself.

Lindsey: This can be very tricky. I once had a boyfriend who had such a low sex drive and it drove me to despair because while his was underactive, it was almost like mine was in overdrive! (Wanting what you can't have, etc.) We navigated it together and talked it over as I had noticed it left me feeling like maybe it was me and maybe he didn't find me sexually attractive. In our case, he had an issue with testosterone so it was a straightforward one to fix. But if the chemistry isn't right, don't waste your time being unfulfilled; it might be time to reevaluate your relationship and really think about what you need to be happy. In another instance, it turned out my partner no longer wanted to be in the relationship and so, of course, that was a huge red flag there! So I suppose it depends on the reason for the differing sex drive, but please don't settle for something if it isn't making you happy. You truly deserve happiness in all aspects of the relationship.

How do I get more confident in voicing what I want sexually?

Lizzy: Sexting! I think it's the best way and how I have often felt the most comfortable starting those conversations. It's easier to be confident behind a screen, so try telling your partner what you would like them to do. Or, if that feels too intimidating, you can always message them and say: "I was just thinking about the other night when you did [insert whatever it was here—no pun intended but take it as you will!], it was so good!" Some positive reinforcement can go a really long way. Sometimes you can find yourself in a situation where your partner will consistently do something you don't like (maybe we can blame porn for this!) and this is where you might need to step it up from positive reinforcement. Something simple like, "I actually prefer it when you do it like this, rather than that." (Code for, "Don't you ever do that to me again, that does not feel good.") It goes without saying that the most gratifying sex you will have is when you can confidently communicate what you want. So if it feels intimidating at first, it will absolutely be worth it!

"You have to communicate and not let anything turn into something that bubbles away and suddenly becomes a lot bigger issue than needed."

Lindsey: You've just got to put it out there. Hopefully, you're with someone you feel you can talk to, someone who respects you and will listen to you and your bedroom needs! Your partner should want to please you as much as you want to please them so if you've got this part sorted the rest will come. Maybe you don't have to use words in the first instance, maybe it's more of a practical guiding exercise! (Lower, lower, to the left, up a bit.)

Afterword

We started writing this book in 2019, before the Covid-19 pandemic began. Even going back and reading one of the opening sentences feels somewhat prophetic: *"Life is unexpected and you just have to roll with it all anyway."* We had no idea how much we would have to live by those words, adapting our lives at an alarming pace that no one would have imagined would be necessary when we saw in the New Year of 2020.

We wrote the majority of this book confined to home, as we all were, willing the people we love to be safe, willing the vulnerable to be cared for, willing this all to end and our lives to feel full and safe again. To the UK's NHS, our Power Rangers! Our absolutely shining lights—without you, we would simply be lost. To the caregivers and frontline workers in any capacity, thank you so very much for everything you have done and continue to do. It is the kindness and grit you have shown that has got so many of us this far.

This global pandemic has taken so much from each and every one of us, in varying degrees of severity, trauma, and hurt. Lots of you will be grieving in very different ways. Grieving the loss of a loved one, the loss of a career, the loss of opportunities and the lifestyle we had all come to take for granted. And to you we send all of our love. 2020: what a shit show. It has put so much of what we have written about here into a new light as it's been such a hard year to sit with your personal battles, however old or new. It's been a year in which lots of people have decided their partner isn't the right one for them or have felt stuck in every aspect of their life as the world seems to resist any attempts you might make to move something forward.

We have both experienced anxiety, doubt, sadness, and worry in boatloads throughout the year. There have been some very lonely parts, where it honestly felt as though your insides are rattling all day long and someone has their foot pinned firmly on your chest. We have all learned to consider our own suffering (which has felt immense) within the context of much greater, collective anguish that both intensifies and diminishes what we have all experienced personally.

Writing this book has been a wonderful distraction and focus for us; it's been the most incredible way to reflect on so many personal moments and milestones in a year when time stood still. We still can't quite believe we've written it. From a sex quip gone wrong, to a podcast, to a book, it's all thanks to you, our glorious readers, that we have been able to undertake this journey together with you. We are most proud of the fact that this has grown from a place of true friendship and love, which we hope this book reflects. What we have shared and ultimately learned from one another has given us the confidence we needed to share it with you. You are incredible and we are very lucky indeed to have a community like you. So thank you, from the bottom of our hearts, for being here, for keeping us going when things got really hard.

How far will we go for love?
Answers

1 *Lindsey*
Very tiring but worth it.

2 *Lizzy*
It didn't get rid of it and just cost me a fortune to be prodded with some tweezers under a microscope.

3 *Lizzy*
I remember it had a lot of Panic! At the Disco on it. I still gave it to him anyway (we did go on to be in a relationship for six years so it wasn't all bad).

4 *Lindsey*
Regretted it the moment it happened and the boy was making power plays to see how far I would go.

5 *Lindsey*
The same boy as question four, what a wanker.

6 *Lizzy*
Don't do this because you then have to be able to keep it up or suddenly snap over it, and it might drive you crazy.

7 *Lindsey*
I won't advocate debt for love but I must admit that I did have a wonderful time.

8 *Lizzy*
I had lots of my first sexual experiences with this boy, all of which were awful really.

9 *Lindsey*
Listen, these are the lengths I will go to.

10 *Lindsey*
Martin didn't say very much.

A few references

Books

Attached: Are you Anxious, Avoidant or Secure?
How the science of adult attachment can help you find—
and keep—love
Amir Levine and Rachel S. F. Heller (Bluebird, 2019)

On Love
Alain de Botton (Grove Press/Atlantic Monthly Press, 2006)

Stay or Leave: A guide to whether to remain in, or end,
a relationship
The School of Life (The School of Life Press, 2021)

The Obstacle Is The Way: The Ancient Art of Turning
Adversity to Advantage
Ryan Holiday (Profile Books, 2015)

The Year Of Magical Thinking
Joan Didion (Harper Perennial, 2006)

ONLINE

Can You Ever Feel "Ready" for Kids?
400 Readers Weighed In
Gyan Yankovich, Repeller.com (07.01.2020)

How To Fail with Elizabeth Day
Elizabeth Day (Host), howtofail, Podcast (2018–),
elizabethdayonline.co.uk/podcast

Acknowledgments

This book means such a lot to us both that we aren't sure where to begin with our big thank yous!

We'll start with our moms, who are second to none and who have shaped the women we are today. For always being proud, and for supporting us in following whatever pipe dream we were onto next.

Lindsey's dad and brother for taking such an interest in it all even though neither are allowed to, or intend to read the book. To Lindsey's boyfriend who probably won't read this book but was there to hold her throughout it all.

Lizzy's family, friends old and new, who all preordered quicker than you can even say "Things You Can't Ask Yer Mom." Lizzy's dad, who had his own personal dream of writing a book that he never had the chance to see become a reality, this wouldn't have been possible without the lessons he passed down while he was still alive. To our friends who never stopped talking about how incredibly proud they were of us throughout this entire process.

Next, we would love to say the biggest thank you to our publishing team at Kyle, for believing in us and this book, even when at our very first meeting we asked for some cookies before we got started. And finally, to our agent Lauren for being so supportive and excited, like our own personal cheerleader, along the way.

LINDSEY HOLLAND

Originally from Stockport, Greater Manchester, Lindsey relocated to London in 2015 to pursue a career as an elderly care physiotherapist within the UK's NHS, curating content for her Ropes of Holland digital channels as a creative outlet, now a full-time focus. Lindsey's natural Northern warmth and humor translates into her carefully curated content, adding personality and engaging her loyal following, contributing to her popularity and success in such a competitive landscape. With her incredible eye for an outfit, Lindsey documents her daily sartorial choices through beautifully shot, authentic imagery. While fashion is a primary focus, she is also passionate about travel, interiors, beauty, and more profound topics such as mental health and relationships. Most recently, Lindsey embarked on a chart-topping podcast series with Lizzy Hadfield, titled *Things You Can't Ask Yer Mum*. The series captures candid conversation between the long-term friends, delving into the intricacies of everything from grief and love to navigating modern dating and sex, offering humorous anecdotes and honest advice.

LIZZY HADFIELD

Hailing from Leeds but now London based, fashion influencer Lizzy Hadfield began her hugely popular blog *Shot from the Street* while studying history of art at the University of Leeds. She soon became a hit with the fashion community, who applauded her for her effortless, relatable approach to styling. She has since created a YouTube channel of the same name. Working with brands including Sergio Rossi, Barbour, and Mytheresa, Lizzy has been named one of the top UK influencers to follow by the *Evening Standard*. She has also featured on Refinery29 and in the *Daily Telegraph*. Lizzy and Lindsey Holland met eight years ago and have since shared their friendship with the world via their podcast *Things You Can't Ask Yer Mum*, offering the advice they so often impart to one another to the rest of the world!